MEANINGFUL CARE

Meaningful Care

A Multidisciplinary Approach to the Meaning of Care for People with Mental Retardation

edited by

Joop Stolk

Department of Special Pedagogics,
Free University,
Amsterdam, The Netherlands

Theo A. Boer

Center for Bio-ethics and Health Law,
Utrecht University, The Netherlands

and

Ruth Seldenrijk

Department of Research and Development,
's Heeren Loo,
Amersfoort, The Netherlands

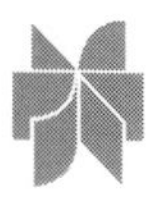

KLUWER ACADEMIC PUBLISHERS
DORDRECHT / BOSTON / LONDON

A C.I.P. Catalogue record for this book is available from the Library of Congress.

ISBN 0-7923-6291-8

Published by Kluwer Academic Publishers,
P.O. Box 17, 3300 AA Dordrecht, The Netherlands.

Sold and distributed in North, Central and South America
by Kluwer Academic Publishers,
101 Philip Drive, Norwell, MA 02061, U.S.A.

In all other countries, sold and distributed
by Kluwer Academic Publishers,
P.O. Box 322, 3300 AH Dordrecht, The Netherlands.

Printed on acid-free paper

Printed in the Netherlands.

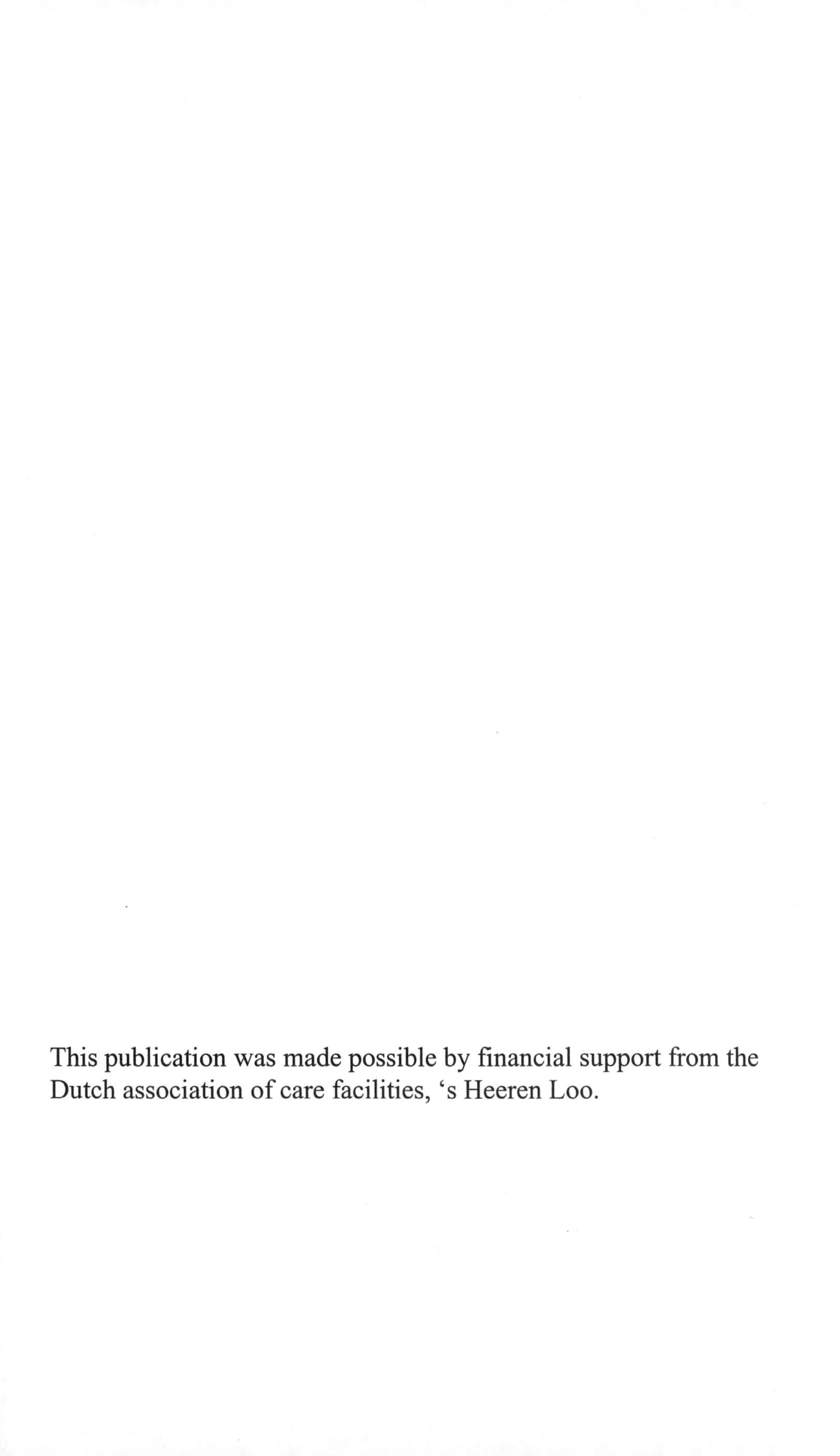

This publication was made possible by financial support from the
Dutch association of care facilities, ‘s Heeren Loo.

TABLE OF CONTENTS

SECTION FOUR - EXPERIENCE OF MEANING IN DAILY CARE

JOOP STOLK, THEO A. BOER, AND RUTH SELDENRIJK[1]

MEANINGFUL CARE

Concepts and Content

1. INTRODUCTION

What makes caring for people with mental retardation meaningful? This question can be looked at from a number of perspectives: what are the experiences of men and women with mental retardation? What kind of experiences of meaning do parents and other relatives have? How can meaning function in daily life and daily care? What is meaningful medical care? What do we, philosophically, mean by "meaning"? How do experiences of meaning of life and meaning of care relate to religious and ideological convictions and perspectives — Christian, Jewish, and Humanistic? And what are the different ethical implications of this all?

However justified all these questions are, meaning of life and meaning of care are indivisible. Any systematic work on the concept, the content, and the implications of meaning in care for people with mental retardation faces the challenge of avoiding compartmentalization and has to be sensitive to the interconnectedness of all the different aspects of meaning. This book is an attempt to meet this challenge. All authors have one thing in common: experience in the care for people with mental retardation. This shared commitment, in combination with different disciplines and interests, yields a volume that intends to provide clues to a comprehensive understanding of what it means to live with mental retardation, and of what it means to be involved in the care for these people.

The contributions of this volume are arranged into four sections: (1) the experience of meaning from a family perspective, (2) the connection between meaning, worldview, and care, (3) meaning in medical care, and (4) the experience of meaning in daily living with people with mental retardation. Before we give an overview of the contents of these sections, we reflect on some terminological questions.

2. TERMINOLOGY

"Meaning"

The concept "meaning" has a variety of denotations in day to day language. A word could have a different "meaning" from one sentence to the next. But if a student misbehaves, and the teacher asks, "what's the meaning of this?", then she is not asking for a definition, but for an explanation of his misconduct. For someone who

Joop Stolk, Theo A. Boer & Ruth Seldenrijk (eds.). Meaningful Care, ix—xv

loves to read, books have "much meaning", whereas for a baby in a crib, books are meaningless. If someone I know well tells me something, I understand him at half a word, but if it is someone from a different culture, I cannot grasp his meaning so easily. In the title of this book, the term "meaning" has more of an evaluative character. Caring for people with mental retardation is meaningful, because it is valuable. Use of the term "meaning" presupposes a value standard, which motivates human actions. In statements such as, "when I care for my kids, I feel happy", or "work means everything to me", people (implicitly) indicate what they consider "valuable" in their lives: caring for children and working hard. That gives "meaning" to their lives. On the other hand, loosing a child or one's job would undermine this "experience of meaning". When parents state that it is meaningful to give of yourself to raise a child with a handicap, they indicate that this giving of themselves is worth it.

That which people consider valuable in their lives is tightly connected to what they try to accomplish in their lives. "We know," states Brümmer, "what the meaning of life is, when we know what dreams and goals to pursue . . . . We know what the meaning of a situation is, when we know what we need to do".[2] Caring for a newborn child is not always easy, because the brand new parents do not know all the ins and outs of the job. Still, they wouldn't think twice about getting up in the middle of the night to feed their child. They find this meaningful, because they know they need to do this, and because they know this crazy schedule is only temporary. They put in the effort with the expectation that their child will grow up to be a healthy individual in a happy family, and will become more and more independent.

It is a different story when a child with a serious handicap is born into a family. Dreams of a happy family are seriously challenged. The parents are shaken up. Raising and caring for their child raises multiple questions. They often don't know what to do. The goal and perspective of their efforts are unclear. This type of situation puts parents under great pressure and they can be overwhelmed with a feeling of meaninglessness. Is the care for their child really worth it?

This example clarifies how the answer to the question about the meaning of parenthood and the meaning of caring for a child assumes a norm (such as health, absence of handicaps, development) and that this norm is based on yet higher norms or ideals (such as making children happy, watching children develop their own personality, etc.). Our experience of meaning is not only determined by norms and ideals, but also by our expectations. There is, according to Brümmer, a tight connection between our actions and our expectations. "It is of little value to strive for an ideal, when we don't expect this ideal to be realized. If we lose faith in the reachability of our ideals, we could easily experience a sense of powerlessness, and ultimately cease striving for these ideals".[3] This is exactly the experience of many parents who have a child with mental retardation. They see their expectations for parenthood vanish into thin air. Their family life is far from what they had imagined. They feel powerless. Their experience of meaning comes under pressure. The birth of a child with mental retardation forces parents into a reorientation of their personal lives and their family life. Expectations have to be adjusted.

"Worldview"

Those who desire to understand the experience of meaning (or lack of meaning) of the parents, must therefore understand the norms, values, ideals, and expectations that move them in life. The most comprehensive framework by which one can interpret the experience of meaning is the worldview of a person. What, then, do we mean by "worldview"? In connection to Holte and Jeffner,[4] we assume that a person's worldview comprises three elements:

1. a cognitive element, i.e., a person's theoretical assumptions about human beings, God, the world, the future of humankind, etc.;
2. an evaluative element, i.e., a person's central valuing system, comprising the values that undergird one's normative ethical convictions, and
3. an affective element, i.e., a person's basic attitudes and feelings towards life. In this manner, theoretical convictions, evaluations and norms, and affections and emotions together establish a person's worldview. A religion, then, is a worldview of which all three elements are characterized by a belief in one (or more) higher power(s).

Our worldview comprises the essence of expectations, convictions, values and feeling used to evaluate our lives. Hence, it directs our lives. In a way, this book can be viewed as a search for underlying worldviews found in the care of people with mental retardation. What is the meaning of their lives? How does the birth of a child with mental retardation influence the parents' experience of meaning? What makes caring for people with mental retardation meaningful?

Meaning: Construed or Found?

Another important terminological question concerns the discussion about the construed versus the discovered nature of meaning in life.[5] One of the key questions is whether or not the reality in which we live has intrinsic meaning or value. One could believe that life is not meaningful in and of itself, but that life's meaning must be attributed. In this option, people give meaning to something or to someone in their life. Meaning, in other words, is created. On the other hand, one could believe that life has an *a priori* meaning, i.e., independent of human experience and valuation. Experiences of meaning, in this option, presuppose that meaning can be unveiled or discovered. People don't create meaning; rather, they discover the meaning of something or someone in their life.

Now if we use this differentiation to look at the life of those who have profound multiple handicaps, there are two possible approaches: either their life has a priori value, in which case others have the task to discover and affirm this value, or their life does not have this value beforehand, and it is up to others to attribute value to their life. In the history of the care of people with mental retardation, one can see how the second approach holds great risks. In the past people with mental retardation did not (and do not) receive adequate care, because they weren't deemed valuable enough.[6] This approach has caused much suffering for people with mental retardation. For this reason, we choose to use the first approach.[7] In this book, we assume that the life of every human being has intrinsic value, including that of those with mental retardation. To express this, we do not speak of "giving meaning", but use the phrase, "experience of meaning". People are not actively, but passively involved in their "experience of meaning".

It is said that Michelangelo once told that his sculptures were already contained in a block of marble, and that all that was left for him to do was to chip off the excessive pieces of marble. The sculpture was there before the artist started working on it, but the artist is necessary to unveil the sculpture. In the same way, the life of a person with mental retardation has meaning before any care-giver enters his life, but in order to discover the meaning of this person's life, it is necessary that he is cared for.

Mental Retardation

As the title indicates, this book is about people with mental retardation. This term is not used by everyone; in some english-speaking countries, the terms "learning disabilities" or "mental", "intellectual", or "developmental disabilities" are customary. Our preference for the term, "mental retardation" matches the terminology used by the American Association on Mental Retardation.[8] This preference, however, is not meant to be dogmatic and, for the sake of variation, other terms will be used as well. Moreover, this volume follows the "people first"-approach and uses therefore the term "people with . . ."

3. OVERVIEW OF CONTENTS

Section One of the volume focuses on the experience of meaning of parents of a child with mental retardation. They are the ones who are most involved with the care. She is their child, "flesh of their flesh". They brought her into the world, cared for her and raised her, with all the care that this brings. Experiences of meaning are existential experiences for parents, as is shown in the contribution by Frances M. Young. She reports on her struggle with questions regarding the meaning of the life of, and of her life with, her son who has mental retardation. Her search leads us to a few key insights into the meaning of caring for people who, through their vulnerability and dependency, confront us with the question about the meaning of our own lives.

In chapter two, Young's experiences are complemented with the results of an empirical research study about the experience of meaning of forty parents who have a child with mental retardation. Joop Stolk and Henk Kars studied the experience of meaning of these parents in relation to their worldview and life history. The results of the study call attention to an aspect of parental coping issues, to which little attention has been paid until now.

In *Section Two*, we take a closer look at the link between the experience of meaning and worldview. Ralph Evers gives an answer from a Jewish perspective, concentrating on the question whether a person's worth is affected by having a mental handicap. Rabbi Evers addresses the position of those with mental retardation in the Jewish community. Although they are not able to follow all the commands of the Halakhah, the Jewish law, it is without question that they are part of God's plan of creation. The meaning of their life is experienced from an eschatological perspective.

Theo A. Boer approaches the question about the meaning of caring for people with mental retardation from a Christian perspective. It is part and parcel of the Christian tradition that every person's life has meaning. To doubt the meaning of life of people with a handicap therefore has a boomerang-effect: when we question the meaning of life of some members of the human community, we are in the process of cutting the branch on which we all sit. The implications for health care are far-reaching. The dominant idea in our culture is that meaning is the result of our own activity. Notions such as "discovering" and "receiving" have moved aside for notions such as "making" and "inventing", as influenced by the Enlightenment.

Hans S. Reinders considers this to be a "transformation in the experience of meaning". He considers this development a threat to the care of people with mental retardation. With this in view, he argues that the quest for meaning is not that important; meaning is experienced as a "by-product" of our lives and actions, and cannot be construed or made a goal in itself. To be sure, he argues, *asking* for meaning may be legitimate. But trying to *answer* the question may cause serious damage, especially to those who cannot build (or choose) meaning into their lives.

Section Three concerns questions about the meaning of medical care. Possibilities in medical and nursing care have greatly increased, especially in the care surrounding the birth of a child. This, in combination with changing views on the value and essence of human life, imposes many complex ethical choices on physicians and parents, in particular parents of a newborn child with mental retardation.

Ruth Seldenrijk explores the possibilities of increasing human well-being, the risks of being ruled by medical technology, and the moral implications of both. His contribution also is an introduction to the next three chapters, which focus in on some specific areas of his contribution.

Technological developments — particularly in the field of genetics — have a large impact on the modern view of man. This, in turn, influences decisions concerning the medical care of children with mental retardation, before and after birth. Ulrich Eibach discusses the moral implications of prenatal diagnostics and selective abortions, when parents are expecting a child with a handicap.

From a practical perspective on paediatric care, Diny van Bruggen highlights questions concerning the meaning, and lack of meaning, of the different forms of medical treatment, with an emphasis on neonatology. She stresses the need for open and comprehensive communication between physicians and parents. Ethicists and physicians play a central role in the public debate about medical-ethical questions concerning the care of people with mental retardation. Comparatively, parents play a relatively insignificant role, while they are the ones most personally involved with questions regarding their child.

In their study on the experience of meaning in the care of children with profound multiple handicaps, Joop Stolk and Henk Kars call upon parents to relate their opinion about abortion as a result of genetic screening and counselling, and on questions concerning non-treatment or selective treatment of children with profound multiple handicaps.

Following this discussion on medical care, *Section Four* focuses on the experience of meaning in the daily care of people with mental retardation. The three contributions in this section contain a critique of the care-concept of some professional care-givers. Sometimes, the person with mental retardation is seen as an object of care rather than as a fellow-man with whom we share our lives. Stanley M. Hauerwas pleads for a radical equality of people with and without a handicap, just as is lived out in the shared-life communities of L'Arche.

According to Pieter A. de Ruyter, meaning of life is experienced in human encounters. On the basis of the experiences of group leaders in group homes for people with mental retardation, he explores the conditions that promote or inhibit human encounters. He comes to the realization that the meaning of life of people with mental retardation is experienced by being open to their unique personhood, by being ready to give and receive, and by having a sincere concern with their existence.

In the last contribution, Joop Stolk analyses the occurrence of serious conflicts in the experiences of meaning of those who provide care to people with mental retardation. For this purpose, he presents a case study in which a care professional seems to have lost all sense of meaning in his care for a boy with mental retardation. The chapter provides criteria and practical clues to dealing with similar crises in the experiences of meaning in caring for persons with mental retardation.

NOTES

1 In 1997, an international conference on the experience of meaning in living and working with people with mental retardation, was held in the Netherlands. The conference was a joint initiative of the Department of Special Pedagogics of the Free University of Amsterdam, the "Vereniging 's Heeren Loo", an organization that provides care for people with mental retardation, and the Christian Association of Care Facilities in the Netherlands. Some of the key contributions presented at the conference were revised and completed with a number of additional texts. This volume contains the result. The Dutch Association of Care Facilities for People with Mental Retardation, 's Heeren Loo provided the necessary funds for this edition, for which the editors are grateful. Moreover, the editors wish to thank Mrs. Marjon Boer for providing the translation of those chapters which were not written in the English language.

2 V. Brümmer, *Theology and Philosophical Inquiry: An Introduction*. London: Macmillan 1981, p. 121.

3 *Ibid.*, p. 131.

4 A. Jeffner, "A New View of the World Emerging among Ordinary People", in G. van den Brink, L. van den Brom and M. Sarot (eds.), *Christian Faith and Philosophical Theology*. Kampen: Kok Pharos, 1992, p. 138. R. Holte, *Människa, livstolkning, gudstro: teorier och metoder inom tros- och livsåskådningsvetenskapen* (Interpreting Human Life and Religious Belief: Theories and Methods in the Study of Worldviews). Lund: Doxa, 1984, pp. 23 ff.

5 See, e.g., R. van Woudenberg, *Gelovend denken. Inleiding tot een christelijke filosofie* (Faith and Reason: An Introduction to a Christian Philosophy). Amsterdam: Buijten en Schipperheijn, 1992.

6 J. Stolk, "The Concept of the Person: Valuing the Life of Severely Handicapped Babies", in J.M. Berg *et al.*, *Report on the European workshop "Bio-ethics and Mental Handicap."* Utrecht: Bishop Bekkers Foundation, 1992, pp. 117-28.

7 Chapter 4, section three, indicates that there are risks involved in the first approach as well.

8 R. Luckasson, D.L. Coulter, E.A. Polloway, S. Reiss, R.L. Schalock, M.E. Snell, D.M. Spitalnik, and J.A. Stark, *Mental Retardation: Definition, Classification, and Systems of Supports*. Washington DC: American Association on Mental Retardation, 1992.

SECTION ONE

EXPERIENCE OF MEANING FROM A FAMILY PERSPECTIVE

FRANCES YOUNG

CHAPTER 1

A PARENT'S SEARCH FOR MEANING IN FAMILY LIFE

1. PERSONAL TESTIMONY: THE CHALLENGE TO FAITH

I grew up in a committed Christian household, and the Christian tradition shaped my understanding of life's meaning. I believed that we were all born for a purpose, and that purpose had to do with moral and spiritual development. Even bad things happened in order to create good people, by trying their mettle, testing their characters.

Later I did a degree in Theology and faced the "problem of evil" with my mind, in other words the questions raised for faith by the presence of suffering and evil in a world supposedly created by a good, loving God. I thought there were reasonable answers, though the case for atheism is not easily dismissed if the problems of sadistic evil and innocent suffering are taken seriously. My simple faith had been challenged. I then married an agnostic, and though still a faithful church attender, became less and less sure in my mind about God and the purpose of life.

Then Arthur was born. Only after quite some months was I told that my difficult baby had severe developmental problems. The placenta had been insufficient and he had been deprived of nourishment and oxygen in the womb — a full-term baby with premature weight and an abnormally small head and brain (microcephalic). The natural distress of an inexperienced mother was compounded by the deep challenge it presented to my already shaky beliefs. I now faced the "problem of evil" not just with my mind but with my heart.

My question was not "Why me?", but "Why do things like this happen at all?" How was I to go on believing in a good Creator, a God with a purpose, when my first-born was apparently unable to develop into an independent person with moral responsibility? It challenged the very heart of my sense of meaningfulness at a deeper level than those earlier theoretical discussions of the "problem of evil". Of course, in a sense it was no different from any other accident. My agnostic husband was able simply to accept the situation as bad luck and get on with coping with it. But it was much harder for me. Faith was not a comfort but a problem.

This was, of course, compounded by the vulnerability of a mother. I had to cope

Joop Stolk, Theo A. Boer & Ruth Seldenrijk (eds.). Meaningful Care, 3—10

with feelings of failure and even guilt, with longing for miracles alongside scepticism about such possibilities, with anxiety about the future and over-possessive attachment to my baby. But it was not just a matter of dealing with the muddled emotions. Hard thinking was essential, so as to reclaim aspects of the Christian story which modernity has largely lost. It was many years before I reached a mature wisdom, wisdom which challenges modern dreams of utopian perfection and enables meaningfulness in terms of creaturely limitation. It is some of the fruit of that long and sometimes arduous pilgrimage which I have been invited to share in this chapter.

What I have to say, then, presupposes Christian faith as the context within which faith desperately seeks understanding and a renewal of meaningfulness. It finds that renewal at the heart of life lived with a person who has severe mental and physical limitations. Arthur is now approaching his 30th birthday. He has no articulate speech and little understanding, he has no self-help skills — we are still feeding him, dressing him and changing his nappies. He has lost what little mobility he had in his teens and even needs assistance to turn over in bed. Yet it is his smiles that minister to me when I return frayed by my professional responsibilities, and others have thanked me for his ministry. His noisy presence in church was the other day described as "Gospel". In other words there is purpose in Arthur's life after all, and he has even generated purpose for others. Several student "Arthur-sitters" have gone on to work with people who have learning disabilities, and my husband after early retirement has devoted himself to working with a number of disability organisations.

So Arthur's life has had purpose even regarded only at human level, but what about those deeper levels of meaningfulness that I have discerned through the challenge and privilege of being Arthur's mother?

2. BEYOND MERE ACCEPTANCE: KEY INSIGHTS

2.1. Corporateness rather than Individualism

Modern societies have become increasingly individualist. In traditional societies people remained rooted in extended families and local communities, doing what their fathers or mothers had done. For the most part we do not. We launch out to find our own way in life. Choice is fundamental. Marriage alliances are no longer arranged but individuals choose congenial partners. Self-fulfilment is the driving force for most of us, even if we have different views of what that fulfilment might be. We find meaning in our personal successes and individual rights.

Yet in doing this we are in danger of losing sight of the fact that it is relationships that make us what we are. Community and corporateness are essential to human thriving and give us a sense of meaningfulness. Of course the Christian faith, which puts a premium on loving one's neighbour, would appear to endorse that, but it is easily taken over by our individualist presuppositions. Instead of valuing what others have to contribute and receiving from them, Christians become activists and do-gooders, thus dominating the situation with oppressive goodwill, and boosting their sense of individual worth. Corporateness requires mutuality.

There are many passages in the epistles of St. Paul which encourage this other perspective. The most obvious perhaps is his image of the church as the Body of Christ, found in 1 Corinthians 12 and Romans 12. In the passage in Romans the emphasis is on each contributing what they have to offer, on gifts like prophecy and service, teaching and charity; but in 1 Corinthians it is about honouring the contributions made by others — even the weakest and least presentable. The body cannot function without having different organs. The eye cannot say to the ear, "You don't belong". By implication the bits of the body we are embarrassed about and cover up are recognised as the most important for the body's functioning.

In the past people have been embarrassed about, and have often hidden away at home or in institutions, those who had mental handicaps. But entering into a relationship with someone who has mental disabilities can be a catalyst for understanding much more profoundly how we all belong to that one body, one humanity. For parents, as distinct from others, this demand to relate is a matter over which they have no choice, but the very real constraints of human existence which they cannot avoid may become a context in which the unrealistic ideals of modern individualism are not only challenged but transcended. The recognition that Arthur's smiles reduce my stress, and that the very simplicity of his extremely earthy needs puts the tensions and politics of University life into fresh perspective, is enough to illuminate that fundamental insight of St. Paul.

Relationships constitute the family. Arthur has siblings and no-one dare ignore the fact that the presence of a severely disabled family member may generate jealousy, hurt, embarrassment, constraints — all kinds of negative forces within family life. We have certainly taken the view that sometimes it is appropriate to leave Arthur in the care of others so as to share with our other children activities we love, like camping, mountaineering or cycling. But this is in order to foster all the relationships in the family. If everyone feels part of it, wanted, loved, affirmed, then a greater sense of corporateness is possible and the contribution and demands of the one who is different can be recognised and integrated. In the early years, play that could involve everybody was a source of family solidarity and hilarity, and established the inclusion of Arthur.

But beyond the nuclear family, it is vital to allow others to be involved. Many years ago I was challenged by a doctor who said, "You think this child is only your responsibility, don't you? It isn't. It is society's responsibility. Society needs handicap." I've spent many years pondering that. Society is certainly, I believe, judged by how it handles difference and disability — its fundamental values are exposed. But if wider society is to be able to respond positively it has to be confronted with it. It is no good if parents and professionals retreat into safe ghettoes. It's never easy, but I am committed to involving Arthur as much as possible in life outside the family, especially church. For people as helpless as Arthur remind us all of our dependence on one another. Indeed one way in which our corporateness may be rediscovered is in recognising our own disabilities. I'm unlikely to forget the experience of saying the general confession week by week with a congregation of people with impaired learning, and discovering that I was no different from them, even if I do happen to be University Professor.

Our corporateness matters. As we noted earlier, according to Paul in I

Corinthians 12, within the body of Christ, the least honourable members are to be the most honoured. It is the experience of the L'Arche communities that people are enriched when they become partners with those who have learning disabilities rather than carers, looking to receive from them and learn from them. Those who have worshipped with people whose mental grasp is limited wonder at the fact that they find themselves infinitely blessed by the gifts of grace received from their uninhibited warmth and simple gratitude, as they share in fellowship and receive the Eucharist.

2.2. Thanksgiving and Receiving

Eucharist means thanksgiving. The moment of real breakthrough for me was when I began to give thanks for Arthur. Arthur became gift not problem. I began to receive from him, and to recognise the extraordinary contribution he had made to shaping the lives of members of the family and indeed of others.

One experience which contributed to this was my renewed call to ordination as a minister. Years before as a student I'd known that if my church had ordained women that's the way my life would have gone. But circumstances had led to a long journey through the wilderness. Meanwhile my church took the decision to ordain women. Suddenly around the time of my 40th birthday, I was driving home from an evening class I'd been teaching. It had gone well and I was on a bit of a high. I stopped at some traffic lights and there came a "loud thought", "You should be a minister". I'm not sure how I drove home. It seemed as if the whole of my life was being presented to me, so that it led up to this call. And at the heart of it was Arthur. He was the gift that fitted me for ministry.

And from there I was led into deepening relationships with people who have learning disabilities. As a student chaplain at the old local subnormality hospital, worshipping with a congregation of almost entirely disabled people, I found that new depth of simplicity in worship referred to earlier. But the greatest debt I owe is to a young man called Francis, a severe epileptic, with whom I travelled to Lourdes. This was years later, in 1991, when Jean Vanier invited me to give a talk on "Spirituality for Parents" at the anniversary pilgrimage of "Faith and Light" (Foi et Lumière). Francis was one of a group from Nottingham, England, with which I shared the journey and the experience from Maundy Thursday to Easter.

It was the evening of Good Friday. We were hearing testimonies from around the world. A man with Down's Syndrome, urged to bring his discourse to an end, said that he must just say what a wonderful mother he had and how he owed everything to her. There wasn't a dry eye in the place, but for me it was like a sword, piercing somewhere deep. I acknowledged all the suppressed guilt about my inadequacies and mistakes in bringing up Arthur, and wept bitterly. Francis comforted me. Then after the meeting we walked round to the holy spring. As a Protestant I'd looked on it more like a tourist than anything else, quite unable to bring myself to go through the motions of touching and venerating as I saw others do. But Francis was an old hand. He took me and with him I climbed off my high horse, simply following the rituals as he did. Then we went to one of the basins and washed each others faces with holy water. My tears and guilt were washed away.

All the significance of my visit to Lourdes I can't share here. But one more insight I must mention. It was at Lourdes that this Protestant came to value even more deeply the figure of Mary as a paradigm of the mother's experience of loss and gift. That insight had come years before at a Carol Service in the local convent chapel. Arthur had been with me in his wheelchair, and a large statue of Mary had overshadowed us. Pushing him home I was given this poem:

Mary, my child's lovely.
Is yours lovely too?
Little hands, little feet.
Curly hair, smiles sweet.

Mary my child's broken.
Is yours broken too?
Crushed by affliction,
Hurt by rejection,
Disfigured, stricken,
Silent submission.

Mary my heart's bursting.
Is yours bursting too?
Bursting with labour, travail and pain.
Bursting with agony, ecstasy, gain.
Bursting with sympathy, anger, compassion.
Bursting with praising Love's transfiguration.

Mary, my heart is joyful.
Is yours joyful too?

There is real loss, real grief for the parents of a child born with mental disabilities. But there's gift too. It's not just a case of acceptance, but of gratitude and thanksgiving.

2.3. Dignity

This business of receiving from persons with disabilities is the key to the issue of dignity. Everything I've said so far about corporateness and gift feeds into what has to be said about dignity and rights.

Everyone, whether able or disabled, needs to make a contribution rather than being the recipient of charity. Value is not something inherent. Even gold has value because human societies have accorded value to it. People are valuable to the extent that they have the esteem and respect of others. Dignity is something we accord each other — our value as individuals rests ultimately in belonging to one another.

There is a tendency in our modern, individualistic culture to think that what matters is rights. The concept of rights is important, of course, in establishing the fact that the oppressed and marginalised have a legitimate stake in society alongside everybody else. But it has become increasingly obvious that there are real difficulties with the concept because of competing rights. To take an example which closely concerns us: Do parents have the right to a peaceful life after the children have grown and flown the nest? Why then are we still, after 30 years, having to find "Arthur-sitters" even to go out for an evening? What about our rights? Rights reinforce individualism, competition, and all the selfish downside of our consumer society. Rights cannot guarantee dignity.

If dignity is to be understood not as something inherent but something we accord one another, then all I have been saying about reciprocity becomes the more important. Carers are not to be conceived as "do-gooders" but as partners. In that partnership there is a two-way process. Carers become friends as they discover their own limitations. Together we learn that what make us human is the capacity to receive help. That insight emerged when a group of theologians met with Jean Vanier to reflect on the L'Arche experience. Another wise saying from that meeting I illuminated by my story about Francis: "My saviour is the one who needs me."

If integrated into so-called "normal" society, there is more chance that persons with disabilities prove catalysts for the discovery of such significant aspects of our humanity. Their dignity lies in their capacity to contribute, and it is vital that we do our best not to "dump" them in homes or push them into their own ghettoes. When I receive the uninhibited embraces of someone with learning disabilities, someone like Pauline, a woman who worships in one of the churches I serve as a minister, I accord her dignity in valuing her and receiving from her, even as I confess my own inadequacies and inhibitions. When I allow Arthur to resolve my stress and anxieties, I am giving him the dignity of a role and the right to contribute.

2.4. The Paradox of the Gospel: an Upside-down World

That role, however, is a long way from conforming to the success-values of our modern culture. Here, as elsewhere, Christian understanding has too often been conformed to modernity. The Gospel is seen as providing health, wealth and success. If you only have enough faith, God will put everything right for you. There has been a resurgence of belief in miracles with the coming of the charismatic movement. This is the mirror-image of the kinds of political idealism that suggests if we can only find the right formula we can put everything right. The mood is encouraged by the successes of modern medicine, our enhanced life expectancy. The Gospels are read with utopian spectacles, but there are unchangeable circumstances, such as incurable disabilities, which not only make it all unbelievable but alert us to other aspects of the Gospel material.

It is worth considering the Beatitudes (Matthew 5.3ff). It is so easy to read them as if they simply promised a future reversal of fortunes: those who mourn will be comforted; those who hunger and thirst will be satisfied. But if we look more carefully we find that the kingdom of God belongs now to the poor in spirit and to those who are being persecuted; and without the mourning and hungering the comfort and satisfaction makes no sense. Beatitudes speak of an upside-down world in which power and success have no place.

A passage from St. Paul which I want to mention in this context is the hymn about Christ, who was exalted by God because he emptied himself, humbled himself and became obedient unto death (Philippians 2. 7-10). The reason that hymn stands in the text is because it provides a model: we are to have the same mind as that, to do nothing from motives of self-fulfilment or success, but in humility to count others better than ourselves. From the standpoint of worldly wisdom this is ridiculous. But divine wisdom is different. Divine wisdom is embodied in Christ. It is foolishness in the eyes of the world (1 Cor. 1.18-25). The success-values of modernity are challenged. Human values are not divine values.

Let's not be sentimental: it is in the anguish of daily care and demands, in the wilderness of protest and frustration, that carers may discover their own inner demons. I'm sure I'm not the only mother to have lost her cool in the middle of the night frantic for sleep, unable to stand any longer the inexplicable screams and howls of her inarticulate child. But it is there also that we reap the harvest of those gifts of the Spirit described by Paul in Galatians 5. 22-3: love, joy, peace, patience, kindness, goodness, faithfulness, gentleness and self-control.

It is an old tradition in the Bible and Christian history that a person meets God in the wilderness. And in the wilderness of distress which is undeniably so often a part of family life with someone with mental disabilities, we may be privileged to discover the depths and the heights within us. Spirituality is too often seen as the individual withdrawing — the flight of the alone to the alone — when self-deception is only unmasked through interaction with others in concrete bodily relationships.

There are significant dimensions to the Gospel which the reality of living with a person with mental disabilities can help to reveal.

2.5. The Cross and Creation

And that brings me to the most important point. At the heart of Christianity is the story of the Cross. It is not a comfortable story — an unjust conviction, an innocent put to death, an incredibly cruel form of execution. It is not enough to see that as just wiped out by the resurrection. Paradoxically for the author of John's Gospel the Cross itself is the hour of glory. Somehow the Body of Christ crucified, the human image of God, embraces all that is defective or "gone-wrong", and transfigures it.

It was in the writings of the French mystic Simone Weil that I came across the idea that creation is an act of abandonment. If God is infinite, nothing else can exist unless God withdraws so as to allow it room. So impairment is inherent in creation. We see it in the leaves of autumn — decay and glory. Limitations are part and parcel of our created existence; death is natural, as is suffering. Nothing is perfect apart from God. This paradox of creation is consistent with the Cross. New life and hope is found in dying, suffering, loss, vulnerability. "Except a grain of wheat fall into the earth and die, it remains alone; but if it dies, it bears more fruit" (John 12.24).

God, according to the Bible, created humanity in the divine image. It is too easy to imagine that the divine image is found in the rationality that distinguishes human beings from animals. For Christians the image of God is seen in Christ. And we are the Body of Christ, not as individuals but as a community. We are, most truly Christ's Body when, like St. Francis we carry the stigmata. Corporately that means, when we are in solidarity with those who live with impairments. They bear the image of the crucified God more obviously than we do.

3. CONCLUSION

My story then is of a journey in faith, from seeing Arthur's condition as a major reason for doubting the goodness, if not the existence, of God, to embracing it as revelatory of what the Christian tradition is all about. I have found that, as in the biblical tradition, the wilderness where we tackle doubts and temptations is the place where we also meet God, and I give God thanks for the special gifts I have been granted through the life of my son. Christianity, someone once said, is not problem-solving but mystery-encountering. Too often we approach the existence of people with mental disabilities as a problem to be solved, as a challenge to meaningfulness. But for me it has been more like revelation, a sacred place, a place of truth.

JOOP STOLK AND HENK KARS

CHAPTER 2

PARENTS' EXPERIENCES OF MEANING

1. INTRODUCTION

The birth of a child who has a handicap is a great disappointment for parents. Their baby does not meet the expectations that they developed during the past nine months. What they value in their lives and parenthood has been tossed in the air. Parents may face emotional problems and difficulties in the upbringing of their child with mental retardation. They may also be confronted with fundamental questions regarding the meaning of life of their child and of their own lives as parents.

A great deal has already been written about the emotional and educational problems of parents.[1] However, little is known about how parents experience meaning. There seems to be a significant gap in our knowledge here. Still, various authors have pointed out how important it is in the assistance of families with a child with mental retardation to pay attention to the questions of parents regarding the meaning of their child's life and the meaning of parenthood.[2] The fact that little attention has been given to this is in part due to the lack of clarity of the term "meaning of life". What is lacking is a description based on the attribution of meaning of parents themselves.[3]

To fill this gap, we conducted a research study about the "experience of meaning" of parents who have a child with mental retardation. We consider the paying of attention to questions about the meaning of the life of a child with a handicap to be of great importance in working with the parents. The purpose of our study is to create greater insight into the nature of these questions and thereby provide a greater understanding of (an aspect of) the coping issues of parents.[4] The study was conducted with parents of children with profound multiple handicaps.[5] We assume that it is especially these parents who are confronted with questions and doubts regarding the meaning of life.

2. RESEARCH QUESTIONS

The research question was developed from the framework of concepts presented in the introduction. The central theme of the experience of meaning of these parents

Joop Stolk, Theo A. Boer & Ruth Seldenrijk (eds.). Meaningful Care, 11—36

can be divided into three sub-themes: how parents experience the meaning of their child's life, the meaning of caring for their child, and the meaning of their own life. These themes are viewed in the context of the worldview and life history of the parents in addition to changes in dominant cultural and societal values. The research question is fourfold:

1. Do parents think the life of their child with profound multiple handicaps has meaning? If so, how do they describe this meaning?
In the first place, the experience of meaning pertains to the life of a child with profound multiple handicaps. Does a child's life have meaning if the possibilities are so limited, if (s)he has so many ailments, if (s)he suffers because of the handicap? The question to the parents is whether they view the life of their child with profound multiple handicaps to be meaningful, whether they doubt the meaning, or possibly don't experience meaning at all.

2. Do parents think that caring for their child is meaningful? If so, how do parents experience meaning in the daily care of their child?
Secondly, the experience of meaning for parents relates to the daily care of their child. This care is burdensome, while purpose and perspective are not always clear. Parents are repeatedly forced to adjust their expectations of the child, or even give them up. This bears consequences for how parents experience meaning. What is the meaning of all their efforts, if their child will never learn to walk, talk, or play anyway, if (s)he will always remain dependent on other people in almost everything?

3. Has caring for their child influenced how parents experience meaning in their own lives? If so, how?
Caring for a child with profound multiple handicaps doesn't leave parents unaffected. This care also influences how they experience meaning in their personal lives.[6] The question asked of parents is whether they have come to look at life differently as a result of caring for their child. In addition, questions were asked regarding norms in the parents' worldviews regarding what is meaningful. What are the most important values in life for parents? What, for them, are the things that "make the world turn"? They were asked whether there is a connection between these values and the meaning they experience in the life of and care for their child with profound multiple handicaps.

4. Has the value that others have placed on the life of children with profound multiple handicaps influenced the meaning that parents experience? If so, how?
When considering the meaning that parents experience, one must look at the effects of the environment, which includes personal (family and friends) as well as societal influences. Given the complex character of this interplay between the individual and its environment, we limit ourselves to the question whether and/or how society's discussion about the prevention of handicaps has influenced parents' experiences of meaning. We focused on the discussion about abortion in the case of expected

handicaps and the selective non-treatment of newborns with profound multiple handicaps. We limit ourselves to the first three questions in this chapter.[7]

3. METHOD[8]

Participants
Forty parents of children with profound multiple handicaps participated in this study. We contacted them via five institutions for people with mental retardation (four group homes and one day care center). The institutions were asked to select parents who would be able to discuss their experience of meaning, who were willing to talk about such a personal and emotionally laden subject, and who (if their child was placed out of the home) still had intensive contact with their son or daughter (at least every other week). The institutions selected 28 sets of parents and two single parents who met these criteria. Eight sets of parents, a father, and a mother, withdrew because they found the subject too difficult emotionally or because their child suddenly fell ill. In the end, 18 sets of parents, 2 fathers, and 2 mothers were open to a discussion regarding their experience of meaning. Together they formed a select group which was not necessarily representative of all parents with a child with profound multiple handicaps. Given the limited purpose of our study, this was not a problem. Our purpose was not to generalize the research results, but rather to give greater insight into the use of the term "meaning" by talking to specific parents who were (emotionally and intellectually) able to exchange thoughts on how they experienced meaning.

The average age of the parents was 44 years and 9 months. They had a relatively high educational level. The fathers all were employed. Most mothers (16) were home-makers. Most of the parents (14 fathers and 14 mothers) had a religious (christian) worldview (70%) and were members of a church community. The remaining parents (6 fathers and 6 mothers) had non-religious worldviews (30%).[9]

The age of the children (19 boys and 3 girls) varied from 3 to 24 years, averaging 15 years and 6 months. In addition to mental retardation, all children had one or more other handicaps. All children had a physical handicap, 7 children were blind, 2 were deaf, and 5 had a seizure disorder. With the exception of one child, none of the children were able to speak. The possibilities for use of alternative communication were limited as well. With exception of 3 children, all children lived in group homes. All parents maintained close contact with their child. In two families, the child with a handicap was the only child. In the remaining families, the parents had (an average of 2) more children. In over half of the families (14), the other children still lived at home.

Procedure
When researching parental experiences of meaning, one is drawn to the personal perceptions of these parents. For this reason, information was gathered by means of in-depth interviews with open-ended questions. The 22 interviews (approximately two-and-a-half hours each) took place at the parents' home. The interviews were conducted by both researchers, who are well experienced with the care of families

of a child with mental retardation.[10]

The interviews were conducted following 30 interview questions, which were derived from the four research questions. The interview with the parents began with a series of questions about their child and their family. During this part of the interview, parents and interviewers got acquainted and developed trust and rapport. This turned out to be significant in the transition to the more personal series of questions about their experience of meaning.

The interviews were tape-recorded and were later transcribed. The parents received a copy of the text with the request to make additions or corrections where necessary. None of the parents made any changes. The interviews were analyzed by both researchers using qualitative analysis methods.[11] The analyses were critically reviewed by two other researchers experienced with qualitative research. Differing opinions were discussed until consensus was reached. The research and the analysis of results were performed in accordance with the criteria for validity (credibility) and reliability (carefulness and neutrality) for qualitative research set by Lincoln and Guba.[12]

4. RESULTS

Based on the four research questions, we now give an overview of the results. The general term, "parents" will be used. This term is used to denote sets of parents as well as the four other parents. Only in cases where opinions differed will we distinguish fathers and mothers. In all other cases, it is assumed that the opinions of both parents were the same. When parents gave more than one answer, all answers were taken into consideration, so that the sum of answers can exceed the number of parents. The results will be illustrated with literal quotes from the interviews. The families will be described using the child's (fictitious) name.

4.1. Experiences of Parents Regarding the Meaning of their Child's Life

Do parents view their child's life to be meaningful? If so, what do parents perceive to be the meaning of life for their child with profound mental handicaps? Interview questions, based on the first research question, were introduced with a question generally framed as follows: "You have told us a lot about your child. It seems as if we already know him a little. You have told us what he can and cannot do. Actually, there is a lot he cannot do. He is seriously disabled. You have also told us how you care for him and what that requires of you. Now imagine an outside person meeting you, and saying: "to be this handicapped, so limited in what he can do, does the life of such a child really have any meaning? Being ill over and over again, sometimes very ill, always needing to be cared for, always remaining dependent . . . His body might be growing, but he is barely developing. He'll never attend school, never be employed, never be involved in a relationship . . . . Does the life of such a child really have any meaning?" We would like to ask you how you would react if someone spoke to you in that way."

a. Parents' Reactions to the Doubts of a Fictitious Outsider

Most parents found this a provoking question that brought them to "the edge of their seats". Five parents stated they would be (very) angry if someone would say such things to them. They would "tell them what it's really like". Two parents thought that there was some truth in the question, but would respond in defense of their child. Two parents could understand the question if it concerned a child that suffered a lot of pain. One parent found it a legitimate question, yet did not agree with it. Most parents (20) would try to erase any doubts by explaining how they see meaning in the life of their child. In the parents' reactions, we found four different argumentations: the life of this child with profound multiple handicaps has meaning a) because (s)he is happy in spite of everything; b) because (s)he means so much to others; c) because the child's life is valued by God; and d) because the child lives and all that lives is meaningful, including the life of those with profound multiple handicaps.

b. Doubts of Others

Along with the doubts of a fictitious outsider, parents were asked if they ever really met someone who voiced doubts about the meaning of their child's life. Over half of all parents (14) say they have never been confronted with that. Two sets of parents say that family members might have had such thoughts, especially in more difficult periods, but have never voiced them. The remaining parents (6) state they have at least once been confronted with the doubts of others, usually strangers.

The parents of Jacco, Peter, and Gary state that they have tasted the presence of doubt in the comments and questions of outsiders. "They find it silly that we visit him every week and that we worry so much. They think we sacrifice our lives too much for him." "Then they say: "look how he's suffering" or, "what kind of life is this anyway . . ." They intend well, finding it too hard for us, and so they worry about us." "After Gary had been in Intensive Care, someone in our family asked, 'wouldn't it have been better not to do it?'" The parents of Tom talk of how their children were confronted on the street with the doubts of others: "neighborhood children said, 'if my mother had had such a child, they would have given it a shot . . .' Luckily our children didn't catch on, because Tom gets tube-feedings, and we always call those tubes 'shots'!"

c. Parents about the Meaning of their Child's Life

Does the life of a child with profound multiple handicaps really have meaning? This question posed by a fictitious outsider provoked a personal reaction in most parents, bringing to mind their own child. The next question is linked to the last one: "what, in your opinion, is the meaning of your child's life?" This wasn't so much a new question as an invitation to parents to, perhaps in different words, describe their thoughts on how they experience meaning in their child's life. This is confirmed in their answers, which are quite similar to their responses to the doubts of the fictitious outsider. All parents find their child's life meaningful. Five reasons stand out in their responses about the meaning of their child's life.

"The life of a child with a handicap has meaning through what (s)he gives to others."
This reason is given the most (11 times). The child's life has meaning because it brings others so much warmth and love. The child who has a handicap is seen as a spring of happiness. "It may sound kind of silly," states Brian's mother, "but I am glad I have him. You see, caring for him can be consuming, but think of the love, the thankfulness and all the things you receive in return from the child. You should see him sitting on his father's lap on Sundays, like a two year old: he loves to hug and cuddle on his lap. Well, you just wouldn't get that from another child . . . what I get from him? A lot! He radiates such warmth and love . . ."

"The life of a child with handicaps has meaning because of who (s)he is."
Eight times, the meaning of the life of a child with a handicap is associated with the (special) "qualities" of the child. His life has meaning, because he is happy, because he is so sensitive to others, because he is so persistent or because of his incredible resilience. For parents, this makes their child's life invaluable and therefore also meaningful. According to his father, John has something that children without a handicap do not have. "They can think, write, and do all sorts of things, but yet they could learn something from John. He knows how to get along with people. He helps one of his blind group-mates with his meals and goes to find a group leader when a resident has a seizure . . . he simply knows what to do . . . he would never hurt a soul. Other people can be so harsh at times . . ."

"The life of a child with a handicap has meaning through how (s)he moves others."
This "reason" is given five times. Living with a child with profound multiple handicaps doesn't leave people cold. Such a vulnerable life softens the heart. It draws others to care and feel love for the child. A child with profound multiple handicaps forces others to think about what is truly important in life. Looking back at Larry's life (he died a month earlier, when a date for the interview had already been set), his mother states: "he stirred up a lot of love in people. Even during the last weeks in the hospital, he would amaze the physicians with his strong will . . . in no time he stirred up something in people who'd notice, "hey, you're a worthy person." Others were filled with tenderness because of the sweetness he radiated. His life was meaningful because he moved others to love him, showing how a person with a handicap truly has much to offer . . ."

"The life of a child with a handicap is meaningful, because God gives life meaning."
Five parents see meaning in their child's life in relation to their faith. The life of their child is meaningful because (s)he was created by God, because the child lives in accordance with God's will, and because in eternity, a life without handicaps awaits the child. In the minds of Ann's parents, every person's life has meaning. "That counts for these children as well, they are created by God. He placed them here. Ann is here, she lives, and as parents you can't just pick up and leave . . . In our society we seem to measure value by 'how much it produces'. That isn't right

. . . The ultimate meaning of her life is that she will be a perfect and complete Ann in heaven . . . that is our comfort. That gives meaning."

"The life of a child with a handicap has meaning because (s)he 'belongs'."
Four parents link the meaning of the life of their child to the relationship (s)he has with others. The child belongs, and can't be discounted, that is why his life is meaningful. Children don't derive their life's meaning from themselves, from what they do or from what they give to others, but through belonging to a community. Stephen's father states, "his existence alone is meaningful. He is one of our children, and this makes you happy, because you have a bond with him . . . Sometimes I say to him, "little buddy of mine." There really is something there between us, perhaps because he says so little and yet we still have this bond . . . He is my oldest son . . . that in itself is meaningful. He is part of your history."

d. Doubts Parents Have about the Meaning of their Child's Life
All parents can identify one or more reasons why their child's life has meaning. We asked parents if there ever were moments when they doubted the meaning of the life of their child.

For fourteen parents, finding meaning in the life of their child has not been an issue. Two of these parents could understand it if other parents have doubts, because the daily care is very strenuous. Art's father contends that parents who doubt the meaning of their child's life are not able to handle their child. His wife adds that this shouldn't be perceived negatively, since the care "really is very strenuous and difficult." His father states, "I can understand it very well, those feelings like 'get me away from this misery, away from this ordeal, away from the stress . . .'"

Eight parents state they do at times doubt the meaning of their child's life. Six parents attribute this doubt to their child's health status: "when he became that ill, the doubts hit me", or, "when the pain was almost unbearable, I thought, 'now it's not worth it anymore.'" Two parents state they only doubted in the beginning, but later on they didn't. They attribute that doubt to the inability to accept their child's handicap: "as long as you ask, 'why,' you're doubting." Ann's mother admits to having had doubts during the time her daughter kept injuring herself. "At those times I prayed, 'well, God, if this is how it's going to be, then please take her home.'" Of course I would have grieved, but I experienced more grief because of . . . how she was. She was in pain, we knew that, otherwise you wouldn't act that way, fear and pain. That you would . . . mutilate yourself like that."

e. Other Points Made by Parents Regarding the Meaning of their Child's Life
Three parents compare the life of their son or daughter with the life of a child without handicaps. The life of such a child is automatically assumed to have meaning. These parents have their questions about that. They conclude that a "healthy" life is not an automatic guarantee for a meaningful life. Even those without a handicap could have experiences in their lives that would make one doubt the meaning of life. Ann's mother gives the following example: "we often say, 'she will never run away from home. She will never get addicted to drugs. She will never

use bad language . . .' We don't worry about what will happen when we're no longer here because there will always be someone to care for Ann . . . My other two girls have a lot of choices and can do a lot. We'll have to wait and see. Anything could happen to them . . . In this world with drugs and prostitution, there are so many terrible things that our children could get involved in . . ."

Two parents point out how the meaning of their child's life partially depends on the quality of the care they receive. Stephen's father has often been surprised that the group leaders see things in a resident that he doesn't see. "Apparently," he states, "meaning is also related to what you discover in a person . . . When a person is less able, meaning is placed more into the hands of what others do with him or her. That meaning lies in the care given to this very limited person. Perhaps it's barely in the person himself, as I see it. To be honest, with regard to some of the residents in Stephen's group I have a hard time speaking of much meaning . . ., someone being so totally in his own world. After all, being human has something to do with communication. The meaning of a person's existence, if you look at the person alone, might be minimal. In those instances it depends more and more on what others do with it. And this person could be placed in a meaningful context . . . To me, meaning has something to do with the humanness of one's surroundings."

4.2. Experiences of Parents regarding the Meaning of their Child's Care

Do parents experience meaning in the daily care of their child? If so, how do they experience this meaning in caring for their child with profound multiple handicaps? What meaning do they find in all their efforts for their child? This second research question was answered by all but three parents. The latter could not indicate if and why the care of their child was meaningful. The question whether the care of their child is meaningful, is answered in the affirmative by the remaining parents. Somehow, caring for their child is worth it.

a. Meaning of Care for the Child

Six parents find caring for their child meaningful because their care contributes to the well-being of their child. For these parents, the meaning, the value of all their efforts, lies in making their child's life as enjoyable as possible. Peter's father is reminded of a bicycle ride with his son. "Last year we vacationed in the province Zeeland. We rode our bicycles through the dunes and among the trees. You can see the sun shining through, and then you're in the shade again. He loves those fluctuations of light and dark. It will often make him laugh." Stuart's father also derives meaning from his son's reactions to the things he and his wife do for him. He tells how Stuart is in especially good spirits during the weekends, when he comes home: "he is home then, in a quiet, relaxed environment. He eats the things he likes, he gets attention, he is active. You can see the enjoyment in his eyes . . . The weekends at home aren't without their difficulties, but all our efforts are apparently worth it."

Ten parents link the meaning of caring for their child with his or her dependence. Is caring for a child with profound multiple handicaps meaningful? "Yes," is the response of these parents, "it is meaningful because the child is so dependent that (s)he wouldn't survive without that care."

Five of these parents find meaning in their efforts as an advocate for their child. Someone has to stand up for their child with profound handicaps. The parents of Jim and Tom state they would "go to battle" for their sons. Art's mother states, "I fight for him when things aren't managed well." His father provides the example of their opposition to the installation of an electronic alarm system on the unit where Art lives.

Four parents link the meaning of caring for their child with their own expertise. Parents are invaluable, since they know their child so well, and for that reason also know just what the child needs. Peter has a difficult time filtering all the stimuli that come his way. As a result, he needs a lot of rest and should never be overstimulated. His parents know this, and are able to inform others (group leaders or a family member that is helping out) about it. Their care is meaningful in that they are able to contribute to their son's well-being through their unequalled experience. For the same reason, Helen's parents had a hard time having their daughter placed. When daily contact with the parents ceases, the parent's expertise also fades (for a large part). "That's why the care doesn't get any better when your child is no longer cared for at home," says Helen's mother.

b. Meaning of Care for the Parents

One parent attributes the meaning of her care (also) to the satisfaction she gets out of it: "it keeps you occupied for hours each day, but it surely isn't time wasted . . . When at night I finally drop down, I really feel fulfilled. At those times I think, 'it might not be easy, but it's worth it.' It may sound crazy, but I wouldn't go without it."

c. Meaning of Care and Basic Values

For three parents, the meaning of care lies in the realization of basic values. The meaning of care springs from the meaning of life.

Helen's parents reiterate how important it is for people to be faithful to each other. The meaning of parents' caring for their children or for their own parents is rooted in their loving care for each other. In this respect, Stephen's father considers the care for children with handicaps as "a test of how humane we are . . . that we treat even the least of human lives with care and respect." Taylor's parents explain how this gives a message to others. If others see how parents relate to their child, then they learn that this life is valuable. The meaning of caring for children with profound multiple handicaps in this case lies in pointing out our responsibilities to each other.

4.3. Parents' Experience of Meaning in Caring for their Child

After being asked about the meaning of the life of their child with profound multiple handicaps and the meaning of caring for him or her, parents were asked a series of questions about the experience of meaning in their own lives, as influenced by their child. First, parents were asked how having a child with a handicap had affected, and still affects, their lives. Did (and does) the child influence their thinking and being; or the choices they have made in their lives? Along this line, parents were asked what they considered important and valuable in their lives, and what, in their opinion, "makes" life; what is life really all about? In their answers to these questions, parents indicated what they considered to be the (ultimate) value of their lives. This value is realized in experiences that are considered meaningful. Parents were asked to give examples of such meaningful experiences from their lives with their child.

a. The Child's Influence on the Lives of the Parents

All the parents indicate that, in one way or another, they are affected by their child with profound multiple handicaps. It is noteworthy that they almost only identify positive effects. Only two parents identify (besides positive effects) some negative effects as well: caring for their child has caused them to be tied to the house (too much) and has hindered their careers.

"The child shaped the character of the parents."

There are various ways in which parents notice how their characters are shaped by the daily care of their child and meeting the child's needs. More than half (12) of the parents noticed this. These parents stated that they have become more patient, calmer, and less hurried, that they have gained more insight into themselves, have become hardier, that because of their child they have truly matured, and have learned how to live with stress.

Caring for a child with a handicap has made Jim's mother a fighter. Especially in her contact with physicians she has learned that ". . . you don't let them brush you off so easily. It matures you in gigantic ways!" Peter's mother states that having a child with a handicap has made her husband "much more confident". His father agrees. He went through a deep valley. Now he feels less vulnerable to other difficulties in life. "You get this attitude of, 'what can be so bad, I've already had to deal with so much.'"

"The child influences the parents' relationships with others."

First and foremost, the relationships within the family are affected. Five parents state that the child brought them closer and strengthened family ties. Brian's mother notices that others sometimes find her too positive when she talks about her son who has a handicap and about the togetherness of her family. "Brian and his older sister are inseparable. She is always there for him. It rarely seems too much: she goes for long walks with him and isn't afraid to change his pants when he is dirty." Jeffrey's father states that he and his wife grew closer: "You always hear about how parents with handicapped children separate. Well, we have had a difficult life together, as our personalities are quite different. You might not always say so, but we did grow closer. You become aware that you need each other and that you don't want to lose the child." Two sets of parents indicate that their marriage survived, but that that it often teetered on the edge. One father says, "there's a point that you're so exhausted that you have nothing left for each other. All the fun is gone . . . There are just worries, worries, worries and the whole world revolves around him (the child with a handicap); that's the only thing you talk about anymore. You just don't get around to each other."

Four parents discuss the effects of having a child with a handicap on their relationships outside the immediate family. Through their child, the parents have got to know people whom they otherwise would have never met. On the other hand, some relationships are broken because of having a child with a handicap. Eight parents state that having a child with a handicap has influenced the way they look at things and relate to others. Paul's mother tells her story: "I don't think I had ever met uncomplicated people before. I didn't know they existed . . . This child simply likes someone; the fact that this person is Jewish or Catholic, young or old, doesn't matter to him. He likes you because you're likeable. He is very honest about that. I think I have adopted some of this simplicity. In any case, I try . . ." Other parents also indicate that having a child with a handicap has led them to relate differently to others. When others face difficulties, it is noticed sooner. Because of their own cares with the child, it is easier to have sympathy for the cares of others. They give their time more freely to be of support to others.

"The child teaches parents to take things into perspective."

More than half of the parents (13) indicate that caring for their child with profound multiple handicaps has helped them develop a better perspective on life. They now can see the value of the things they used to take for granted.

Art's father states: "My son opened my eyes to the relativity of life . . ." He calls to mind an image that has stuck in his memory: the picture of Andrew sitting on the couch next to his uncle, his father's brother. He has cancer. Andrew has profound multiple handicaps. "The one lived 38 years, constantly drinking, an alcoholic . . . Andrew hasn't done a thing, only a faulty family gene inherited from his father and mother . . ." Hans' mother also learned to distinguish the important from the unimportant: "you think more about the things you do . . . You learn to look ahead a little. I don't make a big fuss about the little things that others might get annoyed about and quarrel about. I think it's not worth the fuss. There are worse things, don't get so uptight about stuff . . ."

"The child opens eyes for other values in life."

Taking on a new perspective may result in re-prioritizing your values. Some things which parents used to consider important have taken a lesser place after the birth of the child. On the other hand, they have come to appreciate things they used to pay no attention to. This "turn-about" is identified by eleven parents. Jacco's parents explain how they have, through their son's illness — a serious metabolic disorder —, "come to a better understanding of the essence of life . . ." His father says that "before that time (before Jacco became ill) we used to live according to the motto 'just keep going and all will be fine.' We could handle anything, nothing held us back. We never thought too deeply about stuff . . . we really lived carelessly." Through Jacco, his parents came to see "what makes the world turn: finding happiness around you, being glad in the morning when you get up in good health." Taylor's mother states, "because of him, I've come to appreciate the little things . . . I'm thinking of our grandchildren. When I see them! Goodness, they can stand up just like that! They can eat by themselves! We also are incredibly happy with the little things that show Taylor is progressing . . ."

b. What Parents Find (most) Valuable in their Lives

Parents mostly react positively to questions regarding the child's influence on their lives. They speak of the influence in terms of gain. Caring for their child has shaped their characters, has had a positive influence on relationships, has helped them take things into perspective, and has opened their eyes to other values in life. Parents implicitly indicate what they have come to value: patience, inner peace, standing up for the needs of their child, team-spirit, concern and care for others, ability to take things into perspective, the realization that money isn't everything, etc.

To elaborate on this, parents were asked to describe these values. "What do you consider to be important, perhaps even most important in your life?" "Can you describe what really matters to you in life, what life is truly all about in your eyes?" We limit ourselves to the most frequently occurring responses.

"Happiness (with others)" is the most important value for more than half (12) of the parents. This happiness is experienced in all sorts of ways. For one parent it mostly means "peacefulness at home" and "being home and not having to do anything for a little while." For another parent, the greatest joy is found in the "days we go out with the kids and stop for a little snack." Happiness also means "being appreciated by others." Happiness, some parents say, is "also having something for yourself other than caring for your child," such as a job one day a week, or "working in the yard for an hour or so." Happiness is "enjoying your life together," "working for something together."

For seven parents, "caring for others" is most important. This value is usually associated with caring for people who "have nothing to offer," and who "cannot care for themselves": caring for the elderly, for "lost" youth, addicted to drugs, and above all for people who have a handicap. Life is all about "bringing joy to others," "being glad to give others a chance," and "giving up treasured things for the sake of another."

For four parents, "traits such as honesty, loyalty, and justice" are the most important values in life. For these parents, such values are closely tied to caring for vulnerable and dependent people. Four parents state that for them "faith, the bond with God" is the most important value in their lives. Finally, for two parents "health" is most important in life.

c. Experience of Meaning for Parents in Caring for their Child

Happiness, caring for others, honesty, loyalty, justice, a relationship with God, and health; assuming that experiences of meaning are tied to the realization of these values, parents were asked whether they remembered moments during which they thought: "this is a special moment, surely this is what life is all about." Over half (16) of the parents remember such a moment. During the interviews, it became apparent that these meaningful moments are strongly tied to the personal history of these parents. For this reason, we will not attempt to categorize these experiences. We limit ourselves to a few illustrations of particular moments that parents remember, during which they experienced something of the meaning of their life in relation to their child. In these memories parents share with us what most deeply moves them in life.

"Jeffrey"

Jeffrey's mother explains that she started looking at life completely differently: "I used to think, 'what does it all matter?' We would visit people and then you'd just sit there and chat a little, and later you would think: 'what does it all matter, it seems so pointless.' But when we had Jeffrey, we got to know people who saw life differently. I got more engrossed in books . . . At that time, I discovered that there is a purpose to everything. Nothing happens without a reason. You can learn something from every situation. With everything that comes my way, I ask myself, 'what does this mean for me, what can I learn from this?' I can now enjoy things much easier . . . You hear about people who experience difficult things and ask, 'why me?' Then I think, 'why *not* me?' I mean, so many things happen to people; now it's our turn. I had a handicapped child. So I should learn something from that and then you can start seeing it in a more positive light. Then you don't need to only see it negatively, like you're stuck with a handicapped child; you could learn something from it . . . I think that because of such a child, you see more things around you. This week, we were in a beautiful park, and I love that; on such an occasion, I don't want to see anyone and I just enjoy everything around me, the peacefulness and the birds that are chirping. In the past, I never had time for that and always wanted people around me and to be as busy as possible. I couldn't handle being alone. Now, I love being alone . . ."

"David"

David's parents experience meaning in life in God's care for their child. During the course of the interview they give various examples of this. His mother tells about the worries they have had, and still have, about his health and the difficulties with his feedings. "We have at times stood by his bed and said, 'we just don't know what to do anymore.' Now, he has a gastrostomy tube, but at that time he was still fed orally and it wasn't working. He was so weak and we stood by his bed . . . we were at our wit's end. Then I said, 'why don't we sing, 'God will make a way?'' And he closed his eyes and fell asleep. Yes, it was a miracle . . . Something like that, you never forget."

David has spasticity. He has a hard time fixing his gaze. Once, it came to his parents' attention that he always seemed to look upward. This "looking upward" was seen by the parents as "looking up to God in thankfulness." His mother gives an example. When David is home, she always tucks him in at night, and later checks on him again. "Then he is still awake, and I say, 'mommy and daddy are going to sleep now; are you going to sleep too? I bet you'll sleep really well, won't you?' Then he gives me a trusting look, and looks upward, and I say, 'you're so right: we know that the Lord will care for us tonight.' Then I turn off the light, and you don't hear him anymore, and he falls asleep . . ." For the parents, the "looking upward" of David is the fulfillment of a promise. When he was baptized, the pastor had the congregation sing Psalm 139 verse 7. His father picks up the songbook and reads, "When I consider your wondrous might, I lift up my eyes: I will praise you, my Creator, all my life." When David "looks upward," his parents think of this verse. David cannot talk, but in this way he tells his parents a lot. His mother calls these "beautiful moments."

"Taylor"
Taylor's father is reminded of two moments of "intense happiness." "I believe Taylor infects me with the joy he radiates. It has a contagious effect on me. Such joy, in spite of his handicap; I think it's wonderful! Let me tell you . . . I often ride my bicycle with him, with him in the front. Once, I said to my wife, 'he is so quiet.' 'Yes,' she said, 'he is just staring ahead of him.' Then I said, 'I will whistle something.' So I began whistling and Taylor suddenly started up too. He recognized it and joined me. That makes me so happy. At those times I'm so delighted, and think, 'yes, now we have contact.' Something sparked. It is little things like this . . ." "I remember when he was little. He wasn't interested in anything. But then one time . . . On Saturday mornings this huge truck would drive by from the driver's training school. It always seemed as if Taylor didn't see it . . . Then this one instance something registered. He actually saw the car drive by and followed it with his eyes . . . These are such little things, but you can be endlessly elated by them. I think it is delightful . . . The world opens for him. He joins in with the whistling. He sees a car drive by . . ."

d. Parents regarding the Purpose of Life
During the interviews, the (complex) question regarding parents' experience of meaning was posed from various angles: how has the child influenced the lives of the parents? what do parents find (most) valuable in their lives? what were the moments in which the parents experienced this value, this meaning? Another angle was the linking of the question about meaning to the question about purpose: the purpose of life. Do parents experience a sense of purpose in their lives in general and particularly in the care of their child with profound multiple handicaps?

"The purpose of life is not, or hardly, definable."
Six parents state that they are not sure whether there is such a thing as a purpose of life, and if there were a purpose, they are not aware of it.
Jacco's mother states, "the purpose of our existence? I wouldn't know. No, you just *are*. You try to give it meaning . . . What is meaningful? Well, to see happiness around you, to be joyful. For instance, I'm already happy if I have one good conversation a day with someone. People with mental handicaps are happy when they see you in the morning. If you haven't been there for a week, they say, 'where were you?' Well, you don't hear that too often anymore these days."

For Hans' mother, the primary meaning of life lies in being happy. This, however, doesn't mean that there may not be a higher purpose to life as well, although this may be difficult to discover: "I don't know. I find it very difficult . . . What is the purpose of Hans being that way, and us being this way? I don't know . . . But I think there is more between heaven and earth than we are aware of, but that is about all I can say."

"The purpose of life is found in caring for each other."
For roughly a third of the parents (9), the purpose of life is found in caring for each other, looking out for each other, working on something together. For Beth's father, the purpose of life lies in "making sure that we leave behind a world for our children that is better and somewhat more liveable than it was at the moment we received charge of it . . . and making sure that your children are able to carry on that message and that work in a decent way . . ." Beth's mother agrees with her husband. "That's why," she says, "we have adopted three children in addition to Beth, to pass that on . . ." Patrick's father also emphasizes caring for each other. "What I mean to say is that the purpose of life is not just thinking of ourselves. After all, part of why we're here is to be there for each other."

"The purpose of life seen in relation to God."
The remaining (6) parents see the purpose of life in relation to God. The purpose of life is to "live to honour God;" the ultimate purpose of life lies "in the eternal life with God," in "the new heaven and earth." This life, with illness and handicaps, is seen as temporary. According to Taylor's parents, this has consequences for how they relate to each other. His mother states, "The purpose is: that we were created to fulfill His purposes . . . that we live our lives here on earth as the Lord Jesus lived His. That we therefore are each other's hands and feet and guide in order to magnify and glorify Him. And that others will . . . find [God] through us." This purpose was also fulfilled in Taylor's life. He ended up being the means that brought his brother to God. His father echoes his wife's words. He sums it up in the motto of the Salvation Army: "Saved in order to save." His father brings this into practice in caring for his son and in his volunteer work with drug and alcohol addicts.

e. Experience of Meaning and Worldviews
Along with the question regarding a possible purpose of life came the question of how this relates to the parents' worldview: "Is the way you see meaning in the life of and care for your child related to a certain worldview? Could you say, 'I see it this way, because I have this worldview?'" Most parents interpret this question as referring to a religious worldview, i.e., a religion. This interpretation is reflected in their answers. Unlike the parents with a religious worldview, parents with a non-religious worldview find it difficult to put their worldview into words. Furthermore, there are parents who, although they belong to a church community, do not associate this with what they say about their child and themselves.

In relation to a religious worldview
Relating their experiences to a worldview is most clear for parents who have a

pronounced Christian faith. These parents mostly belong to one of the smaller Reformed denominations or to an evangelical church. A total of seven sets of parents and one father state that their christian faith determines their thoughts about the meaning and purpose of life.

Concerning handicaps and other types of suffering in the world, Stephen's father thinks about the letter of Paul to the Romans in the Bible: "' . . . that the whole creation has been groaning as in the pains of childbirth, and about the futility of life.' It is those things I probably think the most of when I think about Stephen. Wait, I will look it up . . . (he gets a Bible) . . . 'For the creation was subjected to frustration, not by its own choice . . .'[13] You can see that in every area. Just look at politics and at the way different peoples can hate each other. That's why I have never taken the fact that Stephen is so handicapped as a personal punishment. It is a sharing in this common frustration . . . You share in the frustration of a creation in the pains of childbirth, that groans, but with hope . . . that's how I experience it. When I think about the Bible, I don't think about guilt or punishment; rather, you are given a share in that frustration; someone else might get that in unemployment or so . . . I also think that it isn't brought on by some stranger and it isn't the result of a hateful action, that handicap. In that regard I have a certain peace toward God . . ."

When religious worldviews play in the background

For four sets of parents — one father and two mothers —, there also is a relationship with the Christian faith, but it is less outspoken. Their faith plays a 'background role.' These parents belong to one of the larger Protestant churches or are Roman Catholic.

Caring for the children has the first priority in the lives of the parents of Hans. "Your role as a parent is to care for and raise your children in the best way possible." To do this, his parents give it their all. "This," his mother says, "is what we have chosen for." When asked if her worldview plays a role in this, she responds: "perhaps in the background. We are Catholics. That's how we were raised. Let me put it this way, 'you always bring some of it with you.'"

Helen's parents don't see a direct link between experiencing meaning and their worldview. They are members of a church, but it has been more and more difficult to attend because of Helen. Helen's mother: "Her care still claims so much of our lives . . . It feels like I still haven't been able to work on my personal journey . . ." Still, thoughts about God are present in Helen's daily care. Her father: "of course we have thought and looked and searched for how all the pieces fit together. We just haven't figured it out yet. By now we have pretty much dried up spiritually. No, the questions haven't been solved. But our active search we have, I think, put on hold for the last twenty years . . ."

Relationship with non-religious worldviews

Five sets of parents, two fathers, and two mothers see no relationship with their worldview. When probed further, it appears that most of these parents mean to say that they do not have a religious worldview — or not anymore. While talking, there certainly seems to be a relationship to a worldview, but this worldview is difficult to define.

When Jacco's parents try to explain why they work so hard for their son, they do not connect this to their life history, to what they had experienced in the past. Jacco's mother: "well, not from how I was brought up, that I came to be this way . . . Not through religion either. A personal philosophy? Well, simply that you . . . Life is so short. What you have, do something with it, and do it as well as possible."

Beth's parents both have a Roman Catholic background. However, her mother states, "that has had no meaning for me. In our home, we talked much more about war than about religion . . ." She feels a strong aversion toward religious interpretations of the "handicapped life." ". . . It has happened that people said, 'Beth chose to be with you.' That makes me angry. It just isn't true. It is not God who gives you this . . . It can make me really angry; it doesn't seem just. As if there were someone who puts this upon us, upon Beth. As if Beth chose to be handicapped. Then I think, 'this is a logic that just isn't mine, and I don't accept it . . .' It is very simple for me. I just say, 'these things happen' . . . These are things that aren't right. You have to do something about it . . ."

f. Has the Child Enriched the Life of his Parents?

The question series regarding the influence of the child with a handicap on the experience of meaning for parents was ended off with reading a statement. In this statement, parents say that (despite it all) the child with profound multiple handicaps has enriched their life. Parents were asked whether they could find themselves in this statement.

To seven parents this question was not presented. This was mostly because these parents had already given a clear impression that their life is affected positively by their handicapped child. In two cases, the interviewers forgot to bring up the question.

"The child has enriched our life."

Seven sets of parents and two mothers can find themselves in the statement. The life of Jeffrey's parents is enriched through caring for their son. His father paints the picture of a life that creeps along (working, going on vacation . . .), but through Jeffrey he has discovered what it means to care for someone. He has found this an enriching experience.

Larry died a short while ago. Looking back, his parents state that he enriched their lives. His mother, "yes, he enriched our life, he really did . . . material possessions became less important to us. We were happy with him and it is good this way . . . Giving so much love to others through caring for people with mental retardation; they can't be without you anymore, they're afraid to lose you – I love that feeling, how these people love you. If we hadn't had him, we would have never had that experience . . ."

"'Enriched' isn't the right word."

Two sets of parents and three fathers can't immediately agree, and have their objections. "No," says Stephen's father, "enriched is not the right word; you do become more sensitive to certain things, but enriched . . . The richest possession really is a child that is as it was meant to be. I would like to keep it that way . . . I think there is a (big) difference between being healthy and having a handicap; there truly is a rift. I don't think you're a help to the handicapped in denying this rift. They're less capable than we are. That is a fact that shouldn't be denied. You could of course make a virtue of necessity. It does affect you in positive ways, but ultimately you wish you could go and play soccer with the boys."

"A sour expression."
One set of parents and one mother have great difficulty with the word, "enriched". Beth's mother protests against this word usage. "I am sure that if she could speak for herself, she would find it unfair. Sometimes I compare it . . . if Beth had become handicapped later in life, by means of an accident or so, would that enrich your life? My god, it is almost indecent to see it this way!" Helen's parents consider it a "sour" expression. Helen's father: "There is a feeling of sourness when people pretend that it's a beautiful thing . . . It isn't beautiful at all. It might be true in some ways, but if it sounds like 'this is beautiful,' then it isn't true for us."[14]

4.4. Consistency in Use of the Term "Meaning"

In our review of the results of our research, we have thus far limited ourselves to the direct answers of parents to the various research questions. In the conclusion of this chapter, we will assess the consistency of their answers. In closer analysis of the research results, we ask ourselves the following two questions: (a) when parents speak of experiencing meaning in their own life, and the meaning of their child's life, do they have the same denotation for the word "meaning?" (b) Do parents who have similar life experiences of meaning also have a comparable answer to the question regarding the meaning of the life of their child? Both questions address the consistency of parents' experiences of meaning in their own lives and in the life of their child. The first question aims to compare the manner in which they use the term. The second question aims to compare the content of their experiences of meaning.

a. Consistency in the Experience of Meaning: the Nature of the Concept
To determine the consistency of the parents' use of the term "meaning", we proceeded as follows. First, we developed a brief characterization of the experience of meaning in the lives of all the parents. This characterization is based on the parents' statements regarding the purpose of life and on their statements regarding what is (most) meaningful in their lives. All parents' personal lives were greatly affected by the care of their child with profound multiple handicaps. For that reason, in developing a characterization, we also used statements regarding the experience of meaning in the care of their child.

The characterizations are based on selection and interpretation. It is presupposed that meaningful experiences are evidenced in actions that truly matter to those involved. Consequently, we take a parent's answer about experiencing meaning in his or her life as an answer to the question of which actions truly matter to them (a.o. in the care of their child). A characterization of parents' experiences regarding the meaning of their child's life is given in the same fashion. In this case, we look at which actions truly matter in the life of their child, assuming that their child is capable of these actions.

To assure reliability, one researcher, and one person not involved with the study, each independently characterized both aspects of the parents' experience of meaning. Subsequently, the characterizations were compared. At first, this delivered a reliability measure of 87%. After oral deliberations, we were able, with consensus, to make adjustments so that the characterizations were fully in line with each other.

The characterizations of the experiences of meaning in the lives of parents demonstrate that they all conceive this meaning in terms of "actions that truly matter." Life is meaningful when you are happy with each other, when you make others happy, when you care for each other, when you reach out in love, when you help make the world a better place, when you are faithful to one another, when you seek God and walk with Him, etc. In this regard, the answers of parents are in complete agreement.

In characterizing the meaning of their *child's* life, however, only four out of twenty two parents describe this in terms of "actions that truly matter." Paul makes others happy by greeting everyone who walks through the halls of his institution. John helps a blind groupmate with his meal. David glorifies God by thanking Him with a gesture of his head. The father of Stuart is impressed with his son's efforts in being mobile (with all sorts of adaptive equipment). The remaining eighteen parents do not associate the meaning of their child's life with actions. Their child's life has no meaning because of what (s)he does, but through what (s)he is, through what (s)he evokes in others. Rather than in terms of "actions that truly matter," these parents describe the meaning of their child's life by referring to its value. This is even true for the parents of Paul, John, David, and Stuart: in addition to describing meaning in terms of "actions that truly matter," they also describe meaning in terms of the "value of the child for himself and others."

When parents speak of the value of their child's life, they make a distinction between the value of the child's own life and the value of his life for others. A few parents discuss both values. The value of the child's life as discussed by the parents can be subdivided into three types: emotional values, moral values, and religious values.

Emotional values concern the child as well as the parents: "the child arouses positive feelings," "he teaches us to rest and relax," "she is happy," "through him I know what happiness is," "he has fun," etc. A total of fifteen parents find emotional values in the life of their child. *Moral values* are expressed by four parents through statements such as, "he is a person," or "he is here." These "facts" give the child a moral status: his existence gives his life value and makes his life worthy of protection. Another way moral values are expressed are in statements such as, "he teaches us what it means to be a parent," "he prompts others to care for him." The presence of a child with a handicap is an appeal to others to do good. Five parents point to *religious values* in the life of their child: his life is a preparation for a "heavenly life," "a new heaven and earth are awaiting her," etc. Several parents name more than one type of value.

In the various characterizations, it is apparent that the parents use the concept "meaning" differently when discussing their own lives from when discussing the meaning of their child's life. Parents' responses to the question about the meaning of their own lives (including the meaning of *caring* for their child), are in terms of "actions that truly matter." However, their response to the question about the meaning of their child's life is in terms of "the value of their child's life for himself and for others." In addition, four parents speak of the meaning of their child's life in terms of "actions that truly matter."

Why parents make this distinction, is not apparent in the information we have available. One possible explanation might be that the parents solve an existential problem by using this distinction. If they were to use the concept of meaning in the same way for their child's life and for their own life, they would (in most cases) have to draw the conclusion that, because of serious limitations, their child is not capable of "actions that truly matter." This would mean that the child's life has no meaning, that it is meaningless. Since this conclusion would be unacceptable, parents define the concept "meaning" differently in regard to their child's life. In this definition (value of life), it is not presupposed that the person involved is capable of certain activities. The concept "meaning" is not activity-dependent. The child's life has meaning, not through what (s)he can do, but through whom she is and through what her existence brings out in others.

b. Coherence in Experience of Meaning: the Content of the Concept

One possible reaction that parents experience when they have a child with a handicap, is the so-called value-conflict.[15] This conflict develops because the life of their handicapped child does not fit into the worldview of the parents. The birth of a child with a handicap forces parents to re-examine their values. Some parents do this successfully (to a certain point, and after a course of time), while others are not successful and sometimes experience life-long tensions between the experiences of meaning in their own life, and the reality of a life with serious limitations.

The interview data make it possible to investigate whether there are indications that parents experience value-conflicts, and if so, how they deal with these conflicts. We base our analysis on the answers of parents to the question about the purpose of life. Their answers can be subdivided into four categories: (1) for six parents, the purpose of life is difficult, or impossible, to define; (2) for nine parents, the purpose of life lies in caring for each other; (3) for six parents, the purpose of life lies in their relationship with God; and (4) one set of parents is opposed to the idea of a "purpose of life" altogether.

For each category, we evaluate how the answer about the purpose of life is connected to the answer about the meaning of their child's life. When the answers are coherent, there is no reason to assume that there is (at this point in time) a value-conflict. In the presence of discrepancies, we look for clues as to how these are handled by the parents.

"The purpose is difficult to detect."
Six parents state that it is difficult, or even impossible, to indicate what the purpose of life is. This is probably related to their interpretation of the question. The question about the purpose of life is taken as a "commission" to provide a deep, well-rounded view about "life." They are unable, or unwilling, to do this. Evenso, they do answer the question. For them, normal, everyday things take a central position. Life is about being happy with each other; it is about cherishing small things such as the laughter of a child and having time to read the paper. If they value the life of their child in this perspective, there is no conflict: the child is happy and through his presence brings happiness to others.

Jacco's parents state that life is about seeing happiness around you. They are not speaking in big terms. Jacco's mother is happy if she has one good conversation a day. His parents realize, however, that such "happinesses" pass Jacco by. Since he is incapable of relating to others, they wonder if life has any meaning for him. They solve this tension between what they value in life and Jacco's inabilities by reasoning, "and yet . . .", i.e., in terms of a basic trust that there is a meaning, a purpose, and a ground for hope beyond our human doubts and despair. "And yet," the life of their son is meaningful, because others are able to extend so much of their love to him.

Stuart's parents are not sure what the purpose of life is, but they believe that, in any case, it doesn't revolve around material gain. Life's purpose possibly has to do with becoming wise and learning to take things into perspective. They still struggle with the question of the meaning of their son's life. In the middle of this tension, they search for the things that Stuart can, in spite of his handicap, as yet do. With pride, they play a video in which Stuart puts out his fullest efforts to learn how to walk. It is as if they say, "look, despite it all, his life has meaning."

"The purpose of life lies in caring for each other."
For nine parents, the purpose of life lies in taking care of each other, looking out for each other, working on the same goals together. Evenso, they are aware that their child, because of his handicaps, is not able to look out for others. This fact brings none of the parents to the conclusion that their child's life is meaningless. Just as the parents of Jacco and Stuart, they solve this tension between their own values and their child's inabilities by reasoning, "and yet . . ." And yet, the life of their child has meaning, because the child is happy, or because he makes others happy. Some parents realize how vulnerable this happiness is. If their child becomes ill, it could disappear in an instant. They talk from experience when they say that at those times, doubts and questions arise whether (continuing) the life of their child has any meaning left.

"The purpose of life is a relationship with God."
Six parents connect the purpose of life to a relationship with God. The goal is to live a life that honours God. The ultimate purpose of life is eternal life with God in heaven or on a new earth, where handicaps will no longer be.

In the words of three of these parents, there exists no tension between their vision on the purpose of life and how they value the life of their child. As a matter of fact, the opposite is true for the parents of Art. Their child is privileged over others, because "he will be able to enter heaven freely." David's parents are overjoyed to see how the life of their son embodies the purpose of life, namely that a lost person returns to God. Taylor's parents consider themselves "saved by God," and out of thankfulness for this, they seek to serve and save others. Unconscious of his influence over others, their child lives out this purpose in his life. Our conclusion is that these parents have a coherent understanding about life in general and life with serious limitations. We cannot speak of a value conflict in this case.

The remaining three parents in this category are of the opinion that people are called by God to care for one another. The purpose of life lies in answering this call. Confronted with the presence of profound multiple handicaps, these parents realize that their son or daughter will never be able to meet this goal. Does this mean that their child's life lacks meaning? They answer this question in the "and yet . . ." manner: the life of their child is as yet meaningful, because it has other qualities. Tom is sweet and is able to accept things in his life that others never would be able to accept. Through caring for Peter, his parents have gained knowledge of life. The greatest meaning in Ann's life is that there is a new life prepared for her in heaven.

"There is no purpose."

The parents of Jim resist the idea of a "purpose of life." Too many people have pressed them on this issue. Their answer to the question about a worldview leads us to think that their resistance was born out of negative experiences with "people from the church." On the one hand, tones of anger, irritation, and aversion to certain conceptions and people are heard in their reactions, while on the other hand they are proud about the care they give to their son (despite all the opposition and lack of understanding). It is possible to think that the negative feelings aroused by the ideas forced upon them by others have inhibited these parents in their own journey of finding answers to questions regarding the meaning of life.

In our analysis, there appears to be no indication for a value conflict for the parents that we interviewed (at least not in this stage of their life). For seven parents, there was a clear sense of coherence in both aspects of the experience of meaning. For fifteen parents, their statements about the purpose of life do not apply to the life of their child, because it would be impossible for the child to meet this purpose, given his or her limitations. This discrepancy is solved by the parents by an "and yet . . ."-manner of reasoning. There is no indication of a value conflict for these parents either. In the reactions of two parents, we can see that there is a limit to the "and yet . . ."-manner of reasoning. There could be a time when the child suffers to such an extent, that an "and yet . . ." is no longer possible — a time when the meaning of (continuing) the child's life becomes doubtful, since the life of the child no longer meets the purpose of life, as defined by the parents.[16] Whether the experience of meaning for parents regarding their own life or the life of their child is coherent or discrepant, is not connected to the nature of their answer to the question about the purpose of life. Coherency and an "and yet . . ."-manner of reasoning are present both for parents with a strong vision for meaning in life, and for parents who have a difficult time determining the purpose of life.

5. EVALUATION

The purpose of this research study was to create a greater understanding of the experience of meaning of parents who have a child with profound multiple handicaps. We believe this goal has been reached. We looked at parents' experiences of meaning from various angles, asking a series of questions that parents described as relevant and complete in their evaluations. With the results of the research, we would like to conclude with some remarks.

In choosing a research method, we used a type of social science research as our guide, termed "proximity research".[17] This form of research can be characterized by a direct involvement of the researchers with the persons and events within a particular field of research, and by a minimal reduction of the reality of what is being studied. The results of our study confirm that this was the correct choice. Now that the study is over, we realize, even more than before, how much the questions we asked had a personal character. It became apparent that the parents' experiences of meaning were tightly interwoven with their personal history and worldview. For obtaining this sort of information, direct, personal contact with the subjects, preferably surrounded by the safety of their own environment, is essential.

Our choice for a qualitative study with limited quantification fits the picture well. In the data analysis, reduction was avoided as much as possible. In order to get a clear picture of the use of the concept "meaning," we stimulated the parents to do most of the talking. Reactions were only quantified in order to obtain a profile of the (differences between) answers. Thus, a picture of many shades and colours was painted of parents' experiences with meaning, and the use of the term "meaning" was clarified.

Because of the select group of subjects, the research results are not representative for *the* parents of a child with handicaps. It is therefore possible that our study paints too positive a picture of the experiences of meaning of parents caring for a child with profound multiple handicaps. Given the purpose of our study, the lack of representation is not a problem. After all, our goal was not to find representative experiences, but to create a better understanding of the use of the term "meaning" in a particular group of parents. Now that the use of the term "meaning" has become clear in a confined group, a future study with a larger, less select group seems appropriate. We are thinking specifically of parents who have difficulty accepting their child and who are not able or willing to visit their child anymore. It is, of course, not certain whether these parents are willing, or emotionally able, to be involved in such a study.

Both parents and interviewers had a positive appreciation of the interviews. In hindsight, however, there are at least two respects in which this study may have been too limited. First, no attention was paid to the effect time can have on experiences of meaning. While speaking about their experiences, several parents indicated that they used to have different experiences in the past, e.g., because their experiences are strongly related to the health status of their child. Thus, their experience of meaning varies. Had we asked them about their experience of meaning a number of years ago (when their child still lived at home, or when they had difficulty accepting their child), they may have answered differently — and possibly less positively. A follow-up study could focus more on how parents experience meaning over time. Finding meaning is not a static experience. For that reason, possible changes in the experience of meaning over the course of years should be studied in a systematic way. It will be important to find out what brought about these changes. For example, it might be connected with the development of personal insights as influenced by significant events.

Secondly, this study was based on a description of the experience of meaning, which assumed a connection between people's values, actions, and worldviews. This framework determined the structure of the research instrument. Based on this structure, we interviewed parents about their experience of meaning. Looking back, we may have tried too hard to find a tight system connecting beliefs about the meaning of life and the meaning of care. This turned out to be unrealistic. The statements parents made are not so much about *the* meaning of life, but about fragments of their own experience of meaning. Sometimes, experiences of meaning are associated with strong convictions, sometimes they are simply intuitions that are difficult to put into words. Our experience teaches us that one can ask parents about the connection between such things as expectations in life and the experience of the meaning of the lives of their children, but that answers to this question should not be forced. For some, there is only a vague connection; others indicate that they have different values for their own life than for the life of their child. We must leave some room in our questioning and probing for variations in the answers of parents.

A central point in the aid to families of children with mental retardation is assistance to parents in regard to coping with difficulties and questions about raising their child. In the available literature, there is a noticeable gap in information about parental experiences of meaning. Our research therefore focused exactly on this aspect of need often felt by parents. The exact needs of parents, however, are not diagnosed by means of group research. Individual evaluation is needed for this. Naturally, not all parents of children with handicaps need help with coping- and child-rearing issues. Nor would they all want help with experiencing meaning. Our research study does not provide any directions for this. We never asked the parents whether they (ever) wanted professional assistance in this matter. The study does indicate the possibility of parents desiring assistance during a crisis in their experience of meaning, but that their need is not recognized by care-givers. On the grounds of the results of this study, we plead for care-givers to systematically pay attention to the experience of meaning of parents of children with profound multiple handicaps. It should be a regular practice in diagnostic evaluations to assess whether there is a parent need in this respect. A selection of the questions asked of parents in this research study could provide a guideline for discussion with parents regarding their experiences of meaning.

NOTES

1 See, e.g., B.L. Baker, J. Blacher, C.B. Kopp, B. Kraemer, "Parenting Children with Mental Retardation", in N.W. Bray (ed.), *International Review of Research in Mental Retardation*, vol. 20. San Diego: Academic Press, (1997), pp. 1-45; B. Farber, I. DeOllos, "Increasing Knowledge on Family Issues: a Research Agenda for 2000", in L. Rowitz (ed.), *Mental Retardation in the Year 2000*. New York: Springer-Verlag, 1992, pp. 6, 9-84.

2 See K.S. Frey, M.T. Greenberg, R.R. Fewell, "Stress and Coping among Parents of Handicapped Children: a Multidimensional Approach", *American Journal on Mental Retardation,* Vol. 94, no. 3 (1989), pp. 240-9; L. Masters Glidden, "What we do not know about families with children who have developmental disabilities: questionnaire on resources and stress as a case study", *American Journal on Mental Retardation,* Vol. 97, no. 5 (1993), pp. 481-95.

3 Haworth, Hill, and Masters Glidden, and Weisner, Beizer and Stolze researched the influence of religious worldviews on the acceptance of a handicapped child. They are one of the few who mention the parents' experience of meaning. Their study reveals that for parents, their faith may be a means of interpreting and giving meaning to the disability and of interpreting suffering, trouble, and grief. The researchers do not seek to systematically describe the experience of meaning for parents. The central point in their study is the parents' faith as a coping resource. See A.M. Haworth, A.E. Hill, L. Masters Glidden, "Measuring Religiousness of Parents of Children with Developmental Disabilities", *Mental Retardation*, Vol. 34, no. 5 (1996), pp. 271-9; T.S. Weisner, L. Beizer, and L. Stolze, "Religion and Families of Children with Developmental Delays", *American Journal on Mental Retardation*, vol. 5, no 6 (1991), pp. 647-662.

4 Wolfensberger and Menolascino distinguish three types of reactions of parents upon having a handicapped child: novelty shock, reality stress, and value conflicts. Assisting parents with their "value conflicts" implies, they believe, the paying of attention to " . . . the meaning of life and its ultimate values" (p. 484). Our research focuses on this aspect of the coping problems of parents. See: W. Wolfensberger and F.J. Menolascino, "A Theoretical Framework for the Management of Parents of the Mentally Retarded", in F.J. Menolascino (ed.), *Psychiatric Approaches to Mental Retardation.* New York: Basic Books, 1970, pp. 475-93.

5 Since the parents of children with profound multiple handicaps often share the care of their child with professionals (i.e. support workers in day-care centers and special housing facilities) early on, we also included them in our study. In the care of children with mental retardation, they carry a special responsibility, in addition to and with the parents. We asked them, *mutatis mutandis*, the same questions as with the parents. We wanted to know if and, if so, how the experience of meaning differs between parents and support workers. In this chapter, we have to limit ourselves to the parents. For a more detailed report of the entire research study, which includes both the parents and the support workers, see J. Stolk and H. Kars, *Licht en schaduw: Een onderzoek naar de zinervaring van ouders en groepsleiders in de zorg voor kinderen met een ernstige, meervoudige handicap* (Light and Shadow: a Survey of the Experiences of Meaning of Parents and Group Leaders in the Care of Children with Profound Multiple Handicaps). Amersfoort: Vereniging 's Heeren Loo, 1998.

6 The previous contribution of Frances M. Young about "parents in search of meaning in their family life" can be considered a personal development of this theme.

7 The fourth research question will be addressed in section three of this volume (esp. chapter 9) which focuses on Meaning and Medical Care.

8 Given the limited size of this contribution, information about the research method is limited. For more detailed information, see: See J. Stolk and H. Kars (1998) pp. 23-49.

9 These numbers indicate that those with a religious worldview are overrepresented in this survey, as the Yearbook of the Netherlands Central Statistics Agency has found that in 1995, 60% of the Dutch population was member of a denomination, whereas 40% was not. Netherlands Central Statistics Agency, *Statistic Yearbook 1997*. Voorburg: 1997, p. 51.

10 Of the researchers, one has a christian worldview, whereas the other has a non-christian worldview. This mixed background proved to be of considerable value in the interviews.

11 A.L. Strauss and J. Corbin, *Basics of Qualitative Research: Grounded Theory Procedures and Techniques.* London: Sage, 1990.

12 Y.S. Lincoln and E.G. Guba, *Naturalistic Inquiry.* London: Sage, 1985.

13 The Bible: Romans 8:20 (*New International Version*).

14 With reference to the fourth research question, a series of questions followed regarding the influence of society's discussion about the prevention of handicaps on the experience of meaning of the parents. For their reaction, see chapter 9.

15 *Cf.* W. Wolfensberger and F.J. Menolascino, "A Theoretical Framework for the Management of Parents of the Mentally Retarded."

16 Cf. chapter 9, which discusses views of parents concerning the limits of medical care.

17 H. Kars, *Nabijheidsonderzoek. Een visie op praktijkgericht gedragswetenschappelijk onderzoek* (Proximity Research: A Concept of Practice-Oriented Behavioral Studies). Dissertation. Amsterdam: Universiteit van Amsterdam, 1996.

SECTION TWO

MEANING, WORLDVIEW AND CARE

RALPH EVERS

CHAPTER 3

MEANING OF LIFE AND MEANING OF CARE:

A Jewish Perspective

1. INTRODUCTION

Judaism is a religious system, and thus approaches questions about the meaning of life for people with mental retardation from a religious perspective. Even in the oldest sources (Mishna, Oral Studies, 200 CE; Talmud, about 500 CE), people with mental retardation were relieved from all accountability in a civil judicial sense, and, in a religious sense, exempted from having to follow the religious commandments and prohibitions of the Torah (Bible).

Judaism is a religion that focuses on doing good in the *here and now*. It doesn't know a systematic theology. It would be in vain to look for an answer to the question whether a child with mental retardation is created according to *G'd's image*. One could say that the theoretical part of the question whether a person with mental retardation is created in the image of G'd is evidence of a prideful attitude, an egocentrical way of thinking by people who consider themselves healthy: the fact that people with mental retardation fit into G'd's plan of creation, is without question.

People with "normal" mental abilities can have the tendency to feel sorry for people with profound mental handicaps. Rabbi Leib Gurwits, a famous Talmud scholar from Gateshead (northern England), has a completely different outlook on this matter. In his view, this person could very well have a very high *neshama* (soul), and could have been sent to the world to make up for some things that were not attained in a past life. Incidentally, this example shows that the concept of reincarnation is not foreign to Judaism. This soul received a defective body which was not subject to the commandments and prohibitions of the Torah so that he would not be able to do wrong nor commit any transgressions. Rabbi Gurwits describes this person to be very sensitive, to whom others can extend much love by giving him attention and training him in the areas where he does have potential.

Nothing in G'd's creation is accidental or superfluous. A possible goal of human existence is to become G'd's partner in the completion of the Creation. Having a mental handicap makes a person dependent on the (loving) care of his surroundings. The practice of love is one of the pillars that this world is built on, and the measure

Joop Stolk, Theo A. Boer & Ruth Seldenrijk (eds.). Meaningful Care, 39—50

in which this is possible in a society, determines her level of morality.

In spite of his handicap, a person with mental retardation is still a member of the Covenant, and is considered a fellow man who is in need of much care and attention. This answers for a large part the question about the meaning of the care of people with mental retardation.

Judaism is devoted to the study of duties rather than rights. In other words, it is not about which claims people can make on the actions of others, but which actions one should personally take. One of the most important duties in this context is the parents' duty to raise children, a duty that counts just as much for children with a mental handicap as children without such handicaps.

The purpose of raising children is to optimize each of their religious potentials. Even people with mental retardation have a place prepared for them in Gan Eden (Paradise). Although he is different from a person with full mental capabilities, a person with mental retardation is still able to develop a relationship with the Supreme Being. The colour and quality of this relationship are not to be judged by humans.

Although someone with mental retardation is exempted from the commandments, his parents are still obliged to teach him the Torah (Bible) and to raise him in as Jewish a fashion as possible. In child-rearing, one should at all times take into account the individuality and uniqueness of the child. In the context of the care of those who have a mental handicap, this means that it should be provided in a special way, "made to suit."

2. THE DUTY TO RAISE AND EDUCATE CHILDREN

It is the duty of every Jewish parent to teach his children to follow the commandments and prohibitions of the Torah. This is done in order to, as the great scholar Rabbi Shelomo Ben Aderet (1235-1310) explains: ". . . so that he will get used to practising the commandments before he is lawfully of age so that, by the time he comes of age, he is actually capable of following them."[1] It should be clear that parents of a child who is not capable of such responsibilities are exempt from having to raise the child in this manner, since the child could never be expected to practice the commandments and prohibitions, even after coming of age (at age 13 for a boy, and age 12 for a girl).

In addition to the child-rearing duty, there is a duty to teach children about the Torah (Bible). In the Talmud[2], this is traced back to the text, "and you shall teach the words of the Torah to your children."[3] The duty to teach children the Torah is therefore of a Biblical origin, which extends beyond the child-rearing duty which is merely of Rabbinical origin. There are reasons to assume that the father's duty to train his children in the study of the Torah is an intrinsic duty. It is therefore not merely an instrumental duty to prepare children for a life of Torah when they grow up, but it is good in itself.

In his work *Birkat Shemu'el*,[4] Rabbi Baruch Ber Leibowitz, the Rosh Yeshiva of Kaminetz (a Talmud college), proves that the duty to raise a child in the Torah weighs just as heavily as the father's duty to study the Torah himself. The father's duty to hire a teacher to teach his child regarding the Torah is comparable with the duty to hire a teacher for himself, if he cannot study without a teacher. The two duties are two sides of the same coin, two facets of the same mitzvah (command), and they both belong to the personal duties of the father.[5]

Neither the capacities of the father nor those of the child are distinguishable in these commandments. As stated before, the study of the Torah has an intrinsic value which is independent of the question whether it will lead one to accomplish much on intellectual or practical levels. The command to educate children regarding the Torah is only limited by the ability of the child to absorb the lessons.

3. DUTIES OF THE COMMUNITY

Not only the parents, but also the community has the duty to give Torah education to children with a mental handicap, according to the Talmud.[6] There it is mentioned that in old times (about 2100 years ago), Torah training was solely provided by the father: "He who had a father, was taught the Torah by him; he who did not have a father, did not learn the Torah." Rabbi Jehoshu'a Ben Gamla was the first to set up an educational system with a school in every district and town of the Holy Land. All the children had to go to school from the age of six or seven. The Talmud praises Rabbi Jehoshu'a for this initiative, because ". . . without him, the Torah would already have been forgotten." An early authority, the Rama,[7] picks up the thread and proposes that, following the edict of Rabbi Jehosu'a Ben Gamla, the financial burden of educating the youth also becomes the responsibility of the community, so that this responsibility is not left solely to the parents.

The societal duty for financing education was codified by Rabbi Moshe Isserles (1520-1577).[8] If the parents' means are inadequate, the community is obligated to cover the costs of the education. The Tosafists (commentators on B.T. Bava Batra 21a) put forth that a village should only have to appoint a teacher if there are a minimum of 25 students who desire an education. The twentieth century American authority Rabbi Moshe Feinstein (1895-1986) proposes however that children with mental retardation cannot be educated adequately in a class with twenty-five students, and proposes that charity funds be used for the education of disadvantaged children.

The legitimation of the care for people with mental retardation is found in the Jewish vision in the helplessness of the recipient, the respect for all created beings, or in the *Being* of the other in general. Those who are primarily responsible for the care of their handicapped child are the parents. When they are not capable of this, the community takes over the responsibility.

If stated in practical terms, the command would sound as follows: educate people with mental retardation regarding the Torah, raise them in as Jewish a fashion as possible, and support and comfort them. For Jewish parents with handicapped children it is therefore of utmost importance that, when possible, a Jewish care institution is available, since it would offer the best guarantee that the child will receive Jewish care and child-rearing.

4. FULL MEMBERS: THE INCLUSIVE AND THE EXCLUSIVE TENDENCY

We have already concluded that the question of whether people with mental retardation are made in the image of G'd is an erroneous, egocentrical question. To what extent, then, are they considered to be fully accepted members of the traditional Jewish community? The manner in which a community treats her weakest members is after all indicative of the level of moral values and norms in that community.

In Jewish thought, one can distinguish two tendencies when dealing with people with mental retardation. In the *exclusive* tendency, the whole person is defined according to his handicap; (s)he is primarily viewed to be handicapped rather than as a human being. Accordingly, the handicapped person is stigmatized as someone who functions largely outside of the normal rules, which decreases his (sense of) dignity (subjectively), and perhaps even limits who he is as a person (objectively).

The other trend is an *inclusive* tendency, namely, the striving to view the person with a handicap as a regular citizen and to minimalize the disturbance that is brought on by the handicap. In this second view, the handicapped person is basically a normal person who has a problem or handicap. He is not defined or stigmatized as handicapped. At the most, he is excused in those areas where his handicap disables his ability to answer to the daily requirements which society imposes.

My personal interest in this subject was awakened by two children with a mental and physical handicap from abroad who recently lived with us for six years. It was a special experience to see how these children slowly developed in a positive direction. In the beginning, they were unable to communicate with us, and even when they tried, their signals were unintelligible to us. Since their inner world initially was not within our reach, we had to consider them to be mentally retarded.

Various values, norms, and conceptions of the Jewish culture concerned with the range of the handicapped clash with each other. By means of the Halachah (Jewish Law)[9] and the mitzvot (the regulations), the Covenant with G'd becomes a part of the daily lives of individuals and of the community as a whole. In this fashion, the whole of human activity becomes imbued with the G'd-human interaction, which we call "holiness" (kedusha).

In the Jewish religious culture, the occupation with the Torah and the commandments means that one is involved in the most important conversation possible, namely that between G'd and man. It follows that the involvement in the practice of the commandments is a very important matter. As a result, a tension-relationship develops regarding the place of a person with mental retardation: on the one hand the image of G'd, on the other hand not being able to carry on a complete conversation with his Creator. In some cultures, we see a different picture: there, people with mental handicaps are often viewed as spiritually exalted. For example, J. Hes and S. Wollstein point out the large contrast between the Jewish culture and the ancient way of thinking of the Greek culture in which mental handicaps were seen as a source of love, prophecy, and culture.[10] Judaism, in contrast, sees in a mental handicap the antithesis of what the halachic culture admires. The Talmid Chacham (learned) and the Tsaddik (righteous), who closely follow the commandments to the smallest details, and the Chassid (devout) are the heroes of the Jewish culture. They take the ideals of the Covenant seriously, and carry these out with accuracy and great enthusiasm. It is clear that a person with mental retardation could never fit this picture.

5. THE STATUS OF THE BLIND

Following commandments means carrying responsibility; one's duty in this regard includes the fact that the Commissioner assumes one is able. In the Bible, we do not find any explicit references to rules for people with mental retardation. Still, we can discover parallels in discussions regarding the status of the blind in the Jewish Law.

There is a fundamental difference of opinion between two Tanna'im, Rabbi Jehuda and Rabbi Me'ir (2nd century) regarding the extent to which a blind person is obligated to keep the commandments. This difference of opinion has not been solved to this day, despite the age-long discussions. *Rabi Me'ir* basically holds the blind person responsible for all the commandments, but admits that the blind person is exempt from certain commandments that are associated with vision, such as the tri-annual appearance in the temple of Jerusalem during the pilgrimage.

Rabbi Jehuda, on the other hand, exempts the blind person from all prohibitions and regulations of the Torah, independent of the question whether he is capable of keeping them. This general exemption of civil liability is derived from his exemption regarding criminal law,[11] which is a prerequisite for civil liability. Rabbi Jehuda views the blind person as one whole, his handicap determining his whole "legal person". Following the Talmudic discussion, he therefore exempts the blind person from all commandments of the Torah. The background for this conception is explained in the Talmud by Rav Shisha:

> Rabbi Jehuda reasons according to this verse (Deuteronomy 6:1): "Now this is the commandment, the statutes and the judgments which the Lord your G'd has commanded you to learn, that you might do them." He who is subject to the judgments (the civil obligations) is subject to commandments and the statutes (the religious obligations). He who is not subject to the judgments, is also not subject to the commandments.

According to the Talmud, there is therefore a connection between civil judiciary obligations and religious obligations. He who is not capable of carrying the responsibilities of the civil law, is also not kept to his religious obligations by G'd. Partial religious obligations do not exist in Rabbi Jehuda's view; it is all or nothing.

Rabbi Jehuda's thought is not easily explained. A blind person is not incompetent: there are, after all, many commandments and prohibitions that could be kept by a blind person without any difficulties. For this reason, some explain the general disclaimer made by Rabbi Jehuda as a decision by G'd in the Torah which cannot be understood by the human mind. Another possibility is that the Torah exempts people with a (mental) handicap because of their dependent position in regards to other (healthy) people. This, however, does not seem to be a plausible explanation: even children and others who take a dependent position are expected to keep a number of commandments and prohibitions, and for that reason can dependence not be sufficient reason for exemption.

6. IDENTITY SPREAD

Personally, I see a totally different concept worked out in this concept. Before delving into this subject, I will first give a psychological or socio-philosophical inspired explanation, according to an analogy of the so-called "identity spread". Identity spread means that one aspect of the person is viewed as characteristic of the whole. For a handicapped person, this means that his handicap becomes the only basis for his identification on social and religious bases.

Unfortunately, we see this happen all too often. Wheelchair-bound people are often assumed to have mental deficiencies. Some people shout at a blind person, because they assume that he also is hard of hearing. It is not infrequent that people with a handicap are treated as inferior or incompetent. The so-called "does he take sugar?-syndrome" is well-known: questions concerning the handicapped person are addressed to his care-givers or companions. The incidence of the famous violinist Yitschak Perlman, who is seriously handicapped, illustrates this point clearly. While being pushed in his wheelchair into the airplane, the steward asked his companion, "where is *he* going?"

Using the concept "identity spread," we might say that Rabbi Me'ir viewed the blind person as a full person with a handicap, while Rabbi Jehuda views him as a handicapped person in his totality. According to Rabbi Jehuda's view, the handicapped person is, because of his malfunctioning vision, blind in his totality, who can therefore not be held responsible for his actions. One could also explain Rabbi Jehuda's viewpoint as an expression of compassion for the difficult situation of the blind person. Exemption from the commandments signifies the most extreme form of compassion.

At any case, the problem with using an anthropological model is that the meaning of the halachot (regulations and religious-judicial ideas) becomes greatly dependent on human insight, in this case insight in social relations. It emphasizes the creative thought of the human spirit, and denies the halacha as an a-priori structure. An intrinsic connection between the revealed religious system, G'd and the human being, has not been sufficiently explained.

7. HALACHA AS A-PRIORI STRUCTURE OF REALITY

In Jewish thinking, the halacha (Jewish law) precedes reality in the form of an *a-priori* structure. This a-priori structure is the basis of reality, which encompasses all the data of human psychology and also forms the framework of the Torah. Halacha is not only an expression of G'd's will, but in a certain way also of His Essence. A reality permeated by the halacha thus carries an essential relationship with the Creator.

The Torah already existed in a primordial form before the Creation. This primordial halachic system served as a blueprint for earthly reality. The Zohar[12] brings this thought into words as follows: "When G'd created the world, he looked in the Torah and created the world with it."

One can distinguish between the perspective from within (G'd's perspective) and the perspective from without (man's perspective). People tend to see the human world as an independent reality, and attempt to penetrate nature with their limited mental capabilities. Out of an external position, we attempt to impose our psychological and sociological ideas on reality. A completely different approach is the way in which G'd looks at the world from within.

8. ELEVATION OF MATTER

By keeping the commandments and prohibitions of the Torah (Bible), man does not only reach the highest possible level, but at the same time — and this is the essence of the Jewish tradition — he exalts the world around him from a low material level to a higher spiritual level. When man uses his energy in accordance with G'd's will, he reveals the G'dliness in Creation. We are actually speaking here of the victory of the spirit over matter, of form over matter.

Generally, the world is divided into four "realms," namely (inanimate) mass, the flora (the plant world), the fauna (the animal world), and man. Usually, we value plant life over inanimate matter, and animal life over plant life. Man's position is the highest of all, the crown on all of Creation. The greater the measure of vitality in a certain object, the higher its position in Creation. The relative development of the four "realms" is associated with the measure in which the G'dly spark manifests itself at each of these levels. This hierarchy however exists only as viewed from the human perspective. From the G'dly perspective, all things are after all created equal; the same creative power *ex nihilo* imbues all.

9. IMMANENT AND TRANSCENDENT CREATION POWERS

There are two forms of G'dly emanation, which are distinguished in the Kabbala (mystic studies) as *memalle*, the immanent creation power, and *sovev* or *makif*, the transcending creation power. The first creation flood, "memalle", is the G'dly revelation which is covered and obscured to such an extent that it could, as it were, be robed in material and limited matters. This is the G'dly emanation in its revealed form, visible to humanity, which grants created matter existence and life in their final form. The second creation power, sovev, is the eternal G'dly light which is so strong that it cannot be captured in material objects. That is why it is said of sovev that it transcends, or rises above, the created world.

All created matter consists of mass and form. In visible reality, mass and form are inseparable. If we try, however, to separate mass and form in our thinking, than we can say that matter is created by the transcending G'dly power "sovev" or "makif", while form received its appearance by the G'dly emanation, which we call "memalle". The hierarchy in the four "realms" counts only in the perspective of "memalle". In all created matter — from the highest Angel-worlds to our material world —, there is a combination of both sorts of G'dly emanation: a creative, eternal creation power ("makif" or "sovev") not visible by man, and a vitalizing power ("memalle"), i.e., the limited and visible factor in created matter.

The stronger the presence of the vitalizing factor in a certain object, the higher we consider its development. The lower a material creation, the stronger the creative power therein, and the weaker the vitalizing factor. From the perspective of Hashem (G'd), the least developed created beings rise above the more developed creatures, since the primitive creation forms contain more of the eternal creative emanation, which is needed to let them exist.

10. BREAD AS A LIFE CONDITION FOR HUMAN BEINGS

In order to exist, man depends on the lower forms of life on earth, especially from the earth itself. It appears paradoxical that bread keeps the human alive, when to the naked eye, bread takes a much lower place in creation than the human, who houses a G'dly soul. However, since from the beginning of Creation the inanimate matter housed a greater creation power, it is no longer contradictory that all "higher" things are dependent on the earth for their existence. In this light, the worlds of the Torah are easier to understand: "man does not live by bread alone, but man lives by everything that proceeds out of the mouth of G'd."[13] This means that it is not the physical bread which keeps man alive, but the G'dly word or the G'dly power which allows the bread to be the result of a *creatio ex nihilo*. This creating G'dly power is the strongest in inanimate matter or in the plant-realm; this is why man can be kept alive by such means.

In this light, the importance of religious objects in the religious worship service becomes apparent as well. Through the use of material objects, the greatest G'dly revelation in the world comes into being, while at the same time, the religious person reaches the highest form of contact with the Supreme Being.

11. FROM MATERIAL TO SPIRITUAL

The ultimate goal of the creation of this world was that G'd wanted for Himself a "residence in the darkest physical world". This is why the most important task of the Biblical people is to change the material into something spiritual. The human body is made out of opaque material, but the soul has the capability of letting the light shine into the greatest darkness, and is capable of changing the material body into light. This is the most important goal of the creation of man, and of the descendance of his soul into the physical world.

We now return to the conceptions of Rabbi Jehuda, of whom we suggested earlier that he reduces the handicapped person to his handicap. According to the Jewish viewpoint, the commandments have the purpose of changing the physical and earthly into the spiritual. Since a blind person lacks visual ability, he must miss an important part of the world. He therefore also lacks the possibility to exalt the "seen part" of physical reality. Since vision comprises so much, blindness creates an unusual limitation. It is for this reason that Rabbi Jehuda exempts the blind person from the obligation to fulfill the commandments.

From this point of view, the exemption from keeping the commandments is not a case of compassion of our Khaghamim (Sages) with the blind, nor a case of psychological or sociological identity spread. By setting him free from the commandments and prohibitions, we do not debase his personhood as a human being.

12. LACK OF MEANS — LACK OF DIGNITY?

From a human standpoint, we should not view the blind person as a lesser person. Seen from above, however, the blind person lacks the essential instruments in order to exalt an important part of the Creation. Due to his handicap, he does not have eye-contact with the world. This does not mean that he cannot become a faithful servant of the Creator. In many ways, one could compare him to the poor person who does not have money to purchase religious objects (such as phylacteries) and therefore is not able to call up G'dly manifestation in these physical objects.

After this philosophical excursion, we return to the regulating halacha. It is interesting to see how a blind Tanna feels and deals with the halacha. The Talmud talks about Rabbi Joseef, a blind scholar, who initially surprises us by how he uses his handicap as an opportunity to, in a religious sense, feel better than the sighted:

> I used to be in the habit of saying that, when someone told me that the halacha is in agreement with Rabbi Jehuda, who states that a blind person is set free from the commandments, I would make a feast for our Rabbis, since I do keep the commandments even while I am exempted from them.[14]

But this feeling of pride soon makes way for another notion:

> However, I have now heard what Rabbi Hanina has said: "greater is the reward of the one who keeps the commandments while they are obligated to do so, than of those who simply do so out of free will." Therefore, if someone were to tell me that the halacha is *not* in agreement with Rabbi Jehuda, I would make a feast for our Rabbis, because I will receive a greater reward if I keep the commandments while I am obligated to do so.

The responsibility and the duty to keep the commandments is therefore, according to this statement, a measuring tool for human, and especially for religious, dignity.

Later commentators and authoritative sources follow one of the two opinions, although even the followers of the restrictive viewpoint of Rabbi Jehuda still found reasons to oblige the blind to keep the commandments. Maimonides decides according to the conception of Rabbi Me'ir: "the blind are viewed as fully fit business partners in every civil respect." Therefore, after all discussions and considerations — with a few small exceptions — even the blind are kept to all the commandments and prohibitions.

13. THE STATUS OF DEAF AND MUTE PEOPLE

Another parallel we can draw is that of the status of deaf and mute people. In the Mishna (Oral Studies), deaf and mute — as well as mentally incompetent people — are set free from the commandments.[15] One can once again suspect various grounds for the equalization of deaf and mute people with someone who is incompetent in the Mishna. The simplest explanation is usually that a deaf and mute person used to be considered defective and incompetent due to the fact that his inner world was not accessible. He could not tell another person what troubled him, and even when he tried, his signals were generally incomprehensible. He was therefore often considered to have a mental handicap.

At the end of the 19th century, enormous progress was made in the education of deaf and mute people, and for the first time in history, these people learned how to communicate. The fact that deaf and mute people are linked with the mentally incompetent and with minors, makes it plausible to accept that the reason for the exemption was a presupposed mental immaturity.

However, according to the nineteenth century German Rabbi Ezri'el Hildesheimer, this decision in the Talmud was not so much based on the acceptance that a deaf and mute person has a mental handicap, but on the lack of knowledge about what goes on in his inner world, and thus on the lack of insight about his mental capacities. The inability to communicate was apparently the most important problem of deaf and mute people. In the Talmud, the possibility is taken into account that the handicap might correct itself, although this seldom happened. Although the Khakhanim compared the capabilities of deaf and dumb people to those of a minor or a person with mental retardation, they also saw differences between them: in contrast to people with mental retardation, deaf and mute people were allowed to marry and divorce. They based this on a different estimation of their capacities and emotional stability. For deaf and mute people, communication by means of sign language was considered sufficient to carry the necessary formalities to a good end.

While the Khakhamim had insufficient knowledge of the cognitive functioning of a deaf and mute person, they made a global calculation of his societal functioning and assumed, for judicial and religious purposes, a lack of mature mental development. They were nevertheless sensitive to his needs as a human being, even making legal adjustments for this purpose, and arranging marriages and possible divorces for deaf and dumb people.[16] "In the same way in which he is allowed to marry by means of sign language (remieza), he is able to divorce again with use of sign language." The marriage of a deaf and mute person became legalized, because there were no doubts about his ability to develop an emotionally stable relationship with others. Communication by means of signs and lip movements was considered an adequate expression of the will even for simple business transactions. There is some disagreement in the Jewish tradition whether or not lip movements were adequate enough in the case of divorce, since they were more difficult to decipher than sign language. Incidentally, the deaf and mute person was not obligated to follow the commandments and prohibitions.

Rabbi Moshe Feinstein (20th century) explained that there was no "identity spread" in the thinking of our Sages: deaf and dumb people were not completely identified by their handicap. The problem was rather a question of whether it could be assured that sign language and other physical expressions were sufficient for making important decisions.

As stated before, nearly two millennia passed before there was a dramatic change in the nineteenth century. In Vienna, new techniques were pioneered with which deaf and mute people could communicate. Once trained in the new communication techniques, most of the deaf and mute people appeared to have full mental capacities. This new finding led to much discussion among scholars, as a result of which a few leading, eminent Sages wanted to change the status of deaf and mute people. In halachic literature, one can trace both conservative and renewed attitudes.

14. CONCLUSIONS

The Talmudic conceptions regarding the positions of blind and deaf and mute people tell us several things about the meaning of the life and the meaning of the care of people with a mental handicap. We have seen that there are two currents in Judaism: one that seems to exclusively define a person according to his handicap ("identity spread"), and another that views the person with the handicap primarily as a human, be it with some trying limitations. We have contended that it is this latter view which ultimately dominates. This does not take away the fact that, in Judaism, the presence of handicaps is viewed as an impediment to do that for which a human is created and called, namely, to serve G'd by keeping the commandments so that the spiritual can be embodied in the material. The lack of comprehension is an obstacle to knowing the Torah, and the lack of mental competence is an obstacle to keeping the commandments and prohibitions. All this can be interpreted as being an obstacle to being fully human, and therefore as having a strained relationship with the "meaning" of existence. Yet, the existence of people with a (mental) handicap is not meaningless in the least. We have first of all pointed out that people with a mental handicap are in one way or another capable of having contact with the Supreme Being. Moreover, the meaning of everyone's life — and therefore also the life of the person with a mental handicap — is *a-priori* given and is therefore not to be argued. It is on this basis that people with a handicap are full members of the human and religious community.

Concerning the meaning of the *care* of people with a mental handicap, I have contended that Judaism is in the first place a system in which one's duties are defined. The duties of the parent, as well as those of the community, in regards to child-rearing, education about the Torah, and care, are just as much closed to discussion, and so the meaning of the care of people with mental retardation is beyond each and every doubt.

15. EPILOGUE

At the exodus out of Egypt, when the Jews were on their way to the most monumental event in their history — the Revelation on mount Sinai and the giving of the Torah —, all who had suffered Egyptian slavery were liberated. The suffering, the impotence, and the defects were not considered a stigma; rather, it gave the right to freedom.

The blind, the lame, the deaf, the mute, and the person with mental retardation all qualified for G'd's grace. The Covenant at mount Sinai was — it has to be said — however, primarily directed at a nation of healthy people. This does protect us from playing down the existence of mental and other handicaps. The Jewish people were G'd's partner at the foot of mount Sinai. Rabbi Tanchuma emphasizes that the covenant at mount Sinai was made out of a position of physical health and completeness. Rabbi Tanchuma proves that the Jews that stood at mount Sinai were completely restored from their handicaps and defects contracted during their Egyptian slavery:

> How do we know that there were no paralytics among the Jews at the making of the covenant on mount Sinai? Because it was written, "and they stood," which only can mean that they stood on their own feet. How do we know that no one had broken limbs? Because it says, "all what G'd has spoken, we will do." How do we know that no one was deaf? Because it was written, "we will hear." How do we know that no one was blind? Because it was written, "and all people saw." How do we know that no one was mute? Because it says, "all people answered." It is clear, then, that all had been healed from their infirmities.

Physical and mental competency does not imply moral perfection, and does not mean that competent people are capable of functioning without making mistakes. Validity is not equal to moral perfection, but it does help when attempting to develop the highest possible human potential. The Torah and the commandments and prohibitions put high demands upon a person. From a humane and humanitarian viewpoint, this means that a handicapped person is no more and no less a human being than a non-handicapped person, but handicaps do stand in the way of several demands of the halacha (Jewish law).

I would like to finish with the wish that G'd will free us soon from the spiritual darkness of the diaspora, and just as 3310 years ago, He healed all physical and mental handicaps at the Revelation at mount Sinai, this may happen again in the time of the Mash'iach.

NOTES

1 B.T. Megilla 19b.
2 B.T. Kiddushin 29a.
3 The Bible, Deuteronomy 11:19.
4 Kiddushin nr. 27.
5 Shuchan Aruch Joré Dé'a 145:4.
6 B.T. Bava Batra 21a.
7 B.T. Bava Batra 21a.
8 See the Jewish Codex Shuchan Aruch Choshen Mishpat 163:3.
9 For some reading concerning Halachah, *cf.* T. Marx, *Halachah and Handicap: Jewish Law and Ethics on Disability*. Jerusalem/ Amsterdam: 1992-3.
10 J. Hes and S. Wollstein, "The Attitude of the Ancient Jewish Sources to Mental Patients." *Israel Annals of Psychiatry and Related Disciplines,* vol. 2 (1964), pp. 103-16.
11 B.T. Bava Kama 78a.
12 Mystic studies, 2:16.
13 Deuteronomy 8:3.
14 B.T. Bava Kama 87a.
15 Rosh Hashana 3:8.
16 B.T. Jewamot 112b.

THEO A. BOER

CHAPTER 4

MEANING OF LIFE AND MEANING OF CARE:

A Christian Perspective

1. INTRODUCTION

In this contribution, we will review the quest for meaning in the lives of people with mental retardation, and of the meaning of care, in light of what I conceive to be some key concepts of the Christian tradition. This tradition is complex and therefore not always unequivocal. As I will argue, however, the degree of unanimity and consensus is larger than the amount of dissensus.

I commence with some remarks about what we do when we ask questions about the meaning of life, and I will especially point to the action-guiding intention of such questions (section 2). Next, I explore some other theoretical questions, such as whether meaning is formulated "bottom-up," "top-down," or dialectically (section 3). The connection between meaning and experiences of meaning and the question to what degree issues about meaning are different for people with, and without mental retardation, is addressed in section 4. Although all sections are written on the backdrop of a Christian worldview, section 5 addresses the Biblical basis for such an approach more thematically. This chapter ends with some conclusions.

2. INTERPRETATIONS OF THE QUESTION ABOUT MEANING

Some may say that questions concerning the meaning of life are, by definition, misplaced: those who have grasped the meaning of life do not need to raise the question, whereas those who do ask, probably have not grasped the meaning of life. Let us, they might argue, imagine someone who asks for the meaning of nature, of beauty, of love, or of the city of Minneapolis. Who, to put it even more controversially, would ask for the meaning of life of Hispanics, or Caucasians? Is not the sheer fact of their existence proof enough that their lives and existence have meaning?

There are, however, two reasons why questions of this kind may be useful and, to a certain extent, even indispensable. First, many notions about meaning have an action-guiding function, i.e., they explore the possibilities for human response.[1] Let

Joop Stolk, Theo A. Boer & Ruth Seldenrijk (eds.). Meaningful Care, 51—64

us imagine someone asking the question, "is the life of this child with a profound multiple handicap still meaningful?" In case we have no detailed knowledge of the situation, the question can mean a number of different things, such as:

- "What role does God play in the life of this child, and of those he lives with?"
- "Is it preferable to live without a handicap?"
- "Is this child much unhappier than people without such a handicap?"
- "If we had known the risks for this kind of handicap, would we have wanted the pregnancy?"
- "If we had had possibilities for prenatal screening, would there have been reason for selective abortion?"
- "Should we prevent the occurrence of mental retardation, e.g., through genetic counselling, birth-control, personal hygiene, or dietary supplements during pregnancy?"
- "Should we continue to take care of this child?"
- "Should we prevent fetuses with profound mental retardation to be born, if necessary by means of abortion?"
- "Would it under certain circumstances be better to let newborns with a severe handicap die as soon as there is an opportunity?"
- "If this child catches pneumonia, should we treat it?"
- "Can we do anything to make this child happier?"
- etc.

This list of alternatives illustrates that the majority of interpretations of the question have direct or indirect consequences for human action. There is need for orientation, both in evaluating the past ("did we do right?") and in deciding what to do in the future ("which alternatives for action do we have?"). Moreover, these questions tend to pertain not only to actions and attitudes concerning this particular person, but to actions and attitudes towards other people with a similar condition as well. The circle can be drawn even wider: to some, questions about the meaning of life of people with mental retardation may ultimately pertain to the meaning of their own lives, or of life in general. Questions about meaning have built-in elements of prescriptivity and intentionality.[2] This, in turn, means that the way in which questions of meaning are answered, will influence the way in which we treat ourselves and others.

Questions about meaning may serve a second purpose, which can be described as pastoral and/or psychological. When circumstances are difficult, and parents and health care professionals have a hard time coming to terms with the existence of handicaps and suffering, questions about meaning may provide some necessary relief. The opportunity to complain, to verbalize our doubts about the meaning of a situation, a life, or a caring responsibility, may in itself generate strength, motivation, and endurance, apart from any answers or opinions beforehand.

3. MEANING: THE WHOLE AND THE PARTS

It is not surprising that questions about the meaning of a handicap, and the meaning of care, are intertwined with questions about the meaning of *life*, i.e., of the person's entire existence, or even of human life in general. The term "meaning of life" can be compared to the multi-faceted concept of a mosaic: it refers both to the numerous different stones and to the mosaic as a whole. Small, perhaps trivial experiences of meaning, such as a kind remark, a successful working day, a beautiful concert, a prayer, or an experience of nature — or, seen over a longer period of time, health, a happy marriage, a fulfilling job, or a stable family-life — can have self-transcending, sometimes even metaphysical dimensions.

When we recognize that particular elements and experiences of meaning are related to a larger concept of meaning, what direction does this relation take? We can distinguish two alternatives. In a *"bottom-up" relation*, small elements of meaning together constitute larger concepts of meaning which, in turn, may establish an all-encompassing framework of meaning. In this construction, the meaning of a person's life is the sum of a range of down to earth experiences and events, just as a house can be described in terms of the different building materials that were used. In contrast to this, a *"top-down" approach* focuses on the whole. Small events and experiences receive meaning if, and only if, they are part of a larger whole. This can take place in two ways: functionally ("a small event is meaningful only to the extent to which it affirms the whole") or forensically ("a small event is meaningful to the extent to which it is affirmed, or legitimated, by the whole").

Whether functionally or forensically interpreted, a top-down relationship implies that experiences of meaning are not always indicative of reality. Health, prosperity, or a caring responsibility may be *experienced* as meaningful, but when they do not meaningfully and coherently relate to a larger whole (such as a *telos*, a final purpose), they lack real meaning. In this option, experiences of meaning may be deceptive, because they can divert our attention from real needs and perspectives towards trivial, short term goals. Theologically, the larger whole is often referred to as "God," "The kingdom of God," "worship of God," and the like. Such overall ends can also be understood in non-theistic terms, such as communism, a society of autonomous individuals, or a continuing evolution of the human species.

As an alternative to these two approaches to meaning, some assume a more dialectic relationship between the whole and its parts. Smaller events, experiences, and activities add up to a meaningful whole; at the same time, this whole sets the standard of meaning for its parts. In this construction, there is a two-way movement of induction and deduction.[3] To make a reference to the famous ship of Theseus, the whole process of establishing meaning can be compared to building a ship on full sea: there is no safe wharf where engineers can design the ideal ship and subsequently build it. Rather, there is already a vessel of unknown origin, which has to be maintained and further developed in the full turmoils of the ocean.

Assuming a dialectic relationship certainly is attractive: many people find that experiences of meaning contain elements of both; on the one hand, they are rooted in daily life practice while, on the other hand, they are part of an all-embracing framework of meaning. Still, we cannot avoid the epistemological question about the source of meaning, i.e., the question concerning the primary direction of the link between parts and whole. Is the source of meaning in the details, in the actions, in the momentum, in specific events and occasions? Or are the details reflections of a source of meaning which is higher, greater, and more powerful? Who designed and built the ship? If it is a composition of rafts and bars, collected by a mix of experience and coincidence, there is no intended design, and its meaning will be the aggregate of the experiences of its users. If, however, it was built on a wharf from a carefully intended design, its meaning would be given at the onset and the normative basis for using and revising the ship would be found in the drawings.

The reason why all this is important for our reflection on the meaning of life of people with mental retardation is as follows: if life's meaning is the aggregate of the meaning of its parts, we may have to conclude that the lives of people with profound and multiple handicaps are less meaningful than the lives of those with full mental capacities. Compared to people without profound handicaps, some aspects of their lives are damaged or missing altogether. Perhaps there is suffering or pain. There may be serious limitations in development and functioning, the capacities for speech and reflection may be limited, social encounters can be problematic, and there may be less experiences of meaning. If we assume that meaning is composed bottom-up, the presence of profound multiple handicaps may lead to doubts concerning the lives of people with mental retardation, as well as concerning their care.

The alternative — a top-down approach —, however, may imply a risk as well. The assumption that life's meaning is linked to a higher, meaning-giving whole may lead some to conclude — and history has shown that this risk is not imaginary — that the life of people with profound multiple handicaps has less meaning, or no meaning at all. They might argue that the lives of certain people do not fulfill the parameters of what human life is meant to be. Those who do not reflect the Divine intentions for creation, the ends that are inherent to biological evolution, or the rationalistic ideal of the autonomous individual, are at risk to become disqualified. Combined with the fact that ideologies are among the strongest powers that can motivate human beings, a top-down approach may even be more repressive and dangerous than a bottom-up approach.

All depends therefore on the nature of this top-down approach. But there is an alternative which affirms the meaning of the lives of people with profound multiple handicaps just like the lives of anyone else. This alternative is based upon the assumption that meaning is not linked to certain characteristics or capacities, but that meaning is a gift given to every human being, no matter how seriously limited he or she may be.

4. EXPERIENCES OF MEANING

Do we necessarily need to *experience* meaning? The question may be answered rather analytically: meaning must, by definition, in some way be experienced. It is logically impossible that something — a life, an event, a caring responsibility — is meaningful, while at the same time no one involved experiences this. The question is therefore not whether, but by whom, when, and with which intensity meaning should be experienced.

Two remarks should be made. First, people with mental retardation may have experiences of meaning which are less explicit and verbal than those of people with full capacities for verbal expression. Whereas the latter are able to express their experiences by means of statements such as "I like it," "this is very important to me," or "this is worth trying," people with mental retardation will perhaps express their experiences of meaning in a more implicit, non-verbal manner. The absence of explicit verbal expressions does not imply that experiences of meaning are absent. Problems in detecting experiences of meaning in the lives of people with mental retardation may partly go back to the fact that those who raise the question have a highly verbal mindset. To some, it is hard to imagine that experiences of meaning may be contained in other expressions than words and concepts.[4]

All this is not intended to say that people with mental retardation have the same, or nearly the same, experiences of meaning as people without retardation, but that they merely lack the means to communicate about them. It can be argued that some of those who have profound mental retardation have fewer experiences of meaning, that they have experiences of meaninglessness, or that the capacity to experience meaning may even be seriously inhibited.

There is a connection between experiences of meaning and meaning itself, but how tight is this connection? Every human being has moments or periods when experiences of meaning are absent. A person who is unconscious, or someone who is deeply asleep, may lack experiences of meaning. Still, it doesn't seem right to say that their lives *are* meaningless at such moments or periods. Likewise, people in a conscious state of mind may lack experiences of meaning for a shorter or longer period of time. Very few of them would conclude that their lives have become meaningless. Apparently, human beings are capable of bridging gaps of meaninglessness in the hope and expectancy that things are going to be different. Such optimism is based on the assumption that there are prospects for future meaning and that sooner or later experiences of meaning will be back. Hope has a central function here. On the basis of hope, someone who does not experience meaning, may still find the strength to perform certain actions or pursue certain goals.

When a person is not in a position to experience or articulate experiences of meaning, others — parents, spouses, friends, health care professionals — sometimes do this on his or her behalf: hoping, praying, and encouraging. Again, we may take an unconscious state of mind as an example. When a beloved person is in coma, relatives will affirm his or her life's meaning on their behest. But how long can one go on attributing meaning vicariously? In the end, there should be some expectation that the person himself or herself will (re)gain consciousness and will have experiences of meaning him- or herself again. When experiences of meaning are irreversibly absent, there seems to be no point in others articulating or experiencing on his or her behalf. Much depends on the longer term perspectives.

From a Christian perspective, there is an important contribution to make. No human person is irreversibly lost. At the center of the historic Christian creed is the conviction that those who are in Christ will be part of an eternal kingdom of peace and justice in a life hereafter. In that kingdom, "God shall wipe every tear from their eyes; and there shall no longer be any . . . mourning, or crying, or pain."[5] This implies the hope that people with mental or physical handicaps, however severe these may be, not only will see a total recreation of all their human capacities, but will also be able to experience full meaning of life. Instead of sheer dysfunction, suffering, and the prospect of a final and total decay, the Christian believes that suffering will make room for fullness and perfection.[6] However serious mental retardation may be, it is a transient, not a final element of a person's biography. This motivates an inspired and hopeful attitude from others.

Christian faith confesses that meaning is a gift. It is found, recognized and acknowledged rather than made. Life's meaning is inherent to its being-created and is reinforced in its being-redeemed. There may be dialectic elements of meaning as well (small events do contribute to the whole), but the basis for meaning is found in God, not in small events and in human actions. This forensic character of meaning may be critical towards some existing human conceptions about meaning and meaninglessness, according to which subjective human experiences of meaning are the only building stones for larger conceptions of meaning. Some of the other chapters of this volume make clear the lines along which such a critique may go. The polarities between the *humanum* and the *religiosum*, however, need not be exaggerated. Just like most other worldviews, Christian faith vindicates what is human,[7] it tries to find the essence of humanity and it intends to look for what humanity was intended to be. The difference between a Christian approach and many bottom-up contemporary approaches lies in the former's assumption about the all-distorting effects of "sin". The absence of experiences of meaning is seen as a consequence of sin and tragedies which need redemption, rather than as a given fact of life that we can do nothing about. The core of the Christian message is one of hope and reassurance: the lives of human beings have meaning, because their life is part of a larger whole; and insofar as meaning is absent, there are powerful reasons to hope that this is only temporary.

Questions about meaning in the lives, and the care of people with mental retardation may be more poignant and serious than similar questions for other humans, because the presence of suffering leads to doubts whether this life is worth living and whether the care is worth the effort. But the opposite may also be true. People with full human mental capacities sometimes develop doubts about the meaning of life, which might not occur in the lives of people with mental retardation. At the end of the day, it seems, that people with, and people without mental retardation are in the same boat. At certain points or to a certain degree, every human person faces his own imperfections, limitations, and losses. Some day, everyone will lose his independence. Most people fail to meet the criteria of the free, rational individual of the Enlightenment, just like most people do not fit into the description of the healthy, handsome, and happy commercial teenagers. Everyone bridges the gap between ideal and reality. If the life of a person with mental retardation were meaningless because he or she lacks certain attributes of mind or body, any person's life would, to a certain extent, and on certain moments, be without meaning. If caring for people with mental retardation were meaningless, any vocation would be meaningless. When we question the meaning of life of some members of the human community, we are in the process of cutting the branch on which we all sit.

5. BIBLICAL REMARKS

One of the most relevant factors in exploring the Christian tradition is its charter document, Scripture. Does the Bible say anything specific in regard to the meaning of life, and the care of people with a handicap? Of course, *the* Biblical view does not exist. Throughout the Old and the New Testament, different opinions are found. We can identify different lines: a line which sees handicaps as a result of sin and which would not allow people with a handicap to perform sacrificial duties, as well as a line which stresses God's special care for people with handicaps. In the interpretation history of Scriptural texts, both lines have become stressed. Rather than being contradictory, however, these perspectives can be seen as complementing views. Together, they establish the framework for a Biblical view which, as I shall argue, is a basis for compassionate and respectful care.

5.1. Terminology

The terms "retardation", "mental retardation", and "mental handicap" are not part of the vocabulary of the Bible. Clearly, the distinction between mental illnesses and mental retardation was not made as distinctly as is done nowadays. We can assume that mental retardation resided under terms such as "illnesses from birth", "iniquities", "illnesses", and "feebleness". It is possible that people with profound multiple handicaps were referred to as the "poor", "crippled", "disfigured", "blind", "lame", and the like. In the history of Biblical hermeneutics, the "poor in spirit" from the beatitudes in the Sermon on the Mount have often been interpreted as people with limited mental capacities.[8]

5.2. Mental Retardation Part of Creation?

Nowhere in the Bible there is evidence that diseases and retardation are seen as intended parts of human life. Just like scarcity, deprivations, natural catastrophes, and any other causes for human suffering, they run counter to God's good will for his creation. Unlike shadow and light, and cold and warmth (which need each other in order to exist), diseases and handicaps are not an even pair with happiness and health. The rejection of an ontological equilibrium between good and bad separates a Biblical view from religions such as Hinduism and Buddhism, as well as from some of their more westernized variances.[9]

The long history of God and his people as described in Scripture is preceded by the statement in Genesis (the first book of the Old Testament): "and behold, it was very good," and concluded by God's promise in Revelation (the last book of the New Testament): "He shall wipe every tear from their eyes . . . behold, I am making all things new."[10] The history of suffering and failing is put between the brackets of

God's benevolent intentions. No harm experienced on earth was intended to be lasting.

The fact that evil occurs does not mean that God has nothing to do with it, that He is indifferent, or forced to accept its existence out of a lack of power.[11] In the Bible we find examples of natural disasters, illnesses, and deaths, which God seems to use for his purposes. Evil deeds performed by humans, such as the repression of the people of Israel by the Pharaoh, are sometimes made part of God's plan. Despite the fact that God seems to use these events and actions, there are no indications that God wills tragedy and evil, let alone as ends in themselves. In Paul's letter to the Romans, we find the promise that, "to those who love God," "God causes all things to work together for good."[12]

On the basis of biblical stories and experiences, it seems difficult to argue that mental retardation under no circumstance can have anything to do with God's will, i.e., that God is powerless in regard to these and similar tragedies. It is equally hazardous, however, to say anything more than this, because the exact relation of the existence of handicaps to God's will cannot be described abstractly or generally. All we can do on the basis of Scripture and Tradition, is to live in the midst of two dialectically related convictions: handicaps are not part of creation as God intended it, but their existence was not prevented by God.

Because they are not intended as part of God's creation, no one has reason to take the existence of mental handicaps for granted and to demean their impact and severity. Mental retardation is one out of many reminders that something in God's creation went wrong. This fact is vigorously — and painfully — illustrated in the rules connected to worship rituals. According to the Old Testament, those with physical imperfections of whichever nature, were not admitted to perform sacrificial duties:

> No one of your offspring throughout their generations who has a defect shall approach to offer the bread of his God. For no one who has a defect shall approach: a blind man, or a lame man, or he who has a disfigured face, or any deformed limb, (. . .) or a hunchback or a dwarf . . . . No man . . . who has a defect, is to come near to offer the Lord's offerings by fire; since he has a defect, he shall not come near to offer the bread of his God.

Leviticus could not have made it more explicit that handicaps have nothing to do with God; the person who performed sacrificial duties had to reflect God's perfection. But a differentiation is made between the person and his imperfections — a difference which forms the basis for any humane way to treat people with mental retardation. Thus, the person having an imperfection is not rejected from Divine care and grace, for he may

> eat the bread of his God, *both* of the most holy and of the holy, only he shall not go in to the veil because he has a defect, that he may not profane My sanctuaries.[13]

In other words, people with imperfections may not represent God in the Old Testament, but they may certainly share in God's bounties. Only those with contagious diseases, such as leprosy or people with a discharge which might cause infections, are declared unclean and should under certain circumstances be put in quarantine.[14] The exclusion is not based on an evaluation of the value or dignity of these people, but on a medical assessment made by the priest, intended to prevent the spread of diseases and infections.[15] Apart from these exceptions, people with a defect are full parts of the community.

On many occasions in Scripture, God shows a special concern for people with imperfections. In the Old Testament, when speaking about the return of the Jewish people to the land of Israel, God says to Jeremiah,

> Behold, I am bringing them from the north country, and I will gather them from the remote parts of the earth, among them the blind and the lame (. . .). A great company, they shall return here.[16]

In the New Testament, this concern is even more intensified in the mission of Jesus. In Matthew 9:12, Jesus is quoted, saying, "It is not those who are healthy who need a physician, but those who are sick." This is, in a nutshell, what Christianity is all about: to forgive the sins, to restore what went wrong, and to strengthen the weak. One of the most poignant verses which potentially refer to people with mental retardation is found in the Sermon on the Mount:

> Blessed are the poor in spirit, for theirs is the kingdom of heaven.[17]

There is hardly a more powerful way to indicate God's special concern for people with mental retardation than the promise that they will finally inherit the kingdom of heaven.

5.3. Prevention

The assumption that mental retardation is not intended as part of the "good life", is characteristic and highly relevant when compared to some other theistic worldviews. However, passivity — the view that humans can lean backwards because the Creator has meant it this way —, is equally unwarranted as the view that handicaps should be prevented by whatever means. The Biblical conviction that handicaps are a tragedy, provides a stimulus to prevent them just like all other tragedies. Just like there is no point in refusing to take sanitory measures against contamination because God could allegedly prevent diseases, there is no warrant for passivity regarding the prevention of handicaps. Some have argued that many of the Old Testament rules of hygiene, including those for circumcision, not only prevent infections, but also prevent the development of genetic defects. Prevention — yes, but to what price? Unlike the ethical theory of utilitarianism, which defines moral problems in terms of benefits and losses, a Christian ethic does not seek to solve moral problems through a cost-benefit calculus. According to utilitarianism, any sacrifice can be justified as long as the net utility exceeds the harm. A Biblical view precludes such rigorism, because it evaluates ends and means alike. What is at stake, is not whether handicaps should be prevented. The question is: are we justified in pursuing this goal by whatever means, to whatever cost, and to whichever side-effect? What about genetic counselling? Hygienic measures surrounding the process of procreation? Genetic modification? Selective implantation of *in vitro* conceived embryos? Selective abortion after prenatal screening? And termination of life of newborns with severe handicaps?[18] Each and every of these options should be carefully assessed and weighed, without violating the basic value and dignity of people with mental retardation. The main question is not whether or not mental retardation is tragic and should be prevented; it is about the price we pay to achieve this. From a Biblical perspective, we should be cautious not to let tragedy tempt us to sin.

5.4. Sin and Tragedy

In what sense can mental retardation be called "bad" or "evil"? Here, we should make a distinction between two sorts of evil.

Moral evil and its Biblical equivalent, "sin", can be described as a wrong choice of the human will. It can take different forms, such as actions, words, thoughts, and attitudes. It is part and parcel of the Biblical message to try to prevent human beings from the pursuit of moral evil, with the most powerful examples being the Old Testament's Ten Commandments, and the Sermon on the Mount in the New Testament. In fact, most of the Bible is written as an attempt to cope with the reality that human beings can, and do, bring so much evil into the world.

The other form of evil is non-moral evil or tragedy. Non-moral evil can be anything which happens to us which is not the consequence of our own actions.[19] Tragedy can also consist in the fact that we are sometimes confronted with moral dilemmas in which we are forced to choose between two evils.[20]

The two forms of evil can be distinguished. There is, however, as the book of Genesis recounts in the story of the first sin, a link between sin and tragedy. The moral capacity of human beings to pursue good was among the best elements of creation. Adam and Eve were called to bring about happiness, well-being, and development, not only for themselves, but for the rest of creation as well. Their deliberate choice to become disobedient became the beginning of a chain of misery which not only hit themselves, but also the whole creation: pain, hatred, and mortality. Rather than being detectable in single acts and events, however, this causality is general, undetectable, opaque. Except in some circumstances, there is no causal sequence between a particular tragedy and a specific moral offence. At most, the Bible points to sequences of causality in isolated or individual settings.[21]

Why pay attention to this so extensively? Because we sometimes meet the misconception that the birth of a child with a handicap is caused by a sin of the parents, of other relatives, or even of the child itself. In the story about the man born blind, the Gospel of John indicates that the early church rejected such tendencies. When Jesus is confronted with a man who was born blind, his adversaries ask him: "Rabbi, who sinned, this man or his parents, that he should be born blind?" Jesus replies: "It was neither that this man sinned, nor his parents, but it was in order that the works of God might be displayed in him."[22] After this, the man is healed by Jesus; the focus is not on human guilt, but on the Divine benevolence.

5.5. Human Conduct and Attitude

Although handicaps and diseases are not part of the good creation, they are part of human existence. In the Bible, we find a number of rules (more in the Old

Testament than in the New) which apply to human conduct in the face of handicaps and diseases. Why? For the answer, we can refer to the distinction made above: rules are given in order that the existence of tragedies, such as suffering and handicaps, will not tempt us to commit moral evil or sin. Tragedy can make us bitter, or cynical, or even ruthless. This would lead to a vicious circle in which evil would only cause more evil. The presence of a handicap provokes evil in a moral sense when the person with a handicap is treated without respect, benevolence, and justice. In the Old Testament, respect for the disabled is linked to the fear of God: "You shall not curse a deaf man, nor place a stumbling block before the blind, but you shall revere your God."[23] Likewise, "[c]ursed is he who misleads a blind person on the road."[24] In the New Testament, we see that Jesus commits a major part of his earthly ministry to the encounter with people who are sick, blind, or poor, and those who for other reasons have become excluded. He meets each one of them as bearers of full human value and dignity.

Diseases and handicaps may function positively, i.e., as a means of bringing people together, as a means of triggering moral concern, as a source for finding true compassion, and as a stimulus to finding what is really meaningful and valuable; in short, they may be a means of "displaying the works of God".[25] Handicaps can unite and separate, they can bring sensitivity and they can paralyse, they can reinforce moral concern and they can cause us to escape from our moral duties. Albeit this could be one answer to the question for meaning in the lives of people with mental retardation, it should be stressed that we never know the *purpose* of a handicap. Talking about the meaning of a handicap can only be done in terms of "making the best of it", so we can speak of meaning only in a secondary sense: in the best case, this tragedy can be a factor which stimulates people to become better people; in the worst case, the opposite will happen.

There might be another, secondary, effect: handicaps may give people without such a handicap a clearer view of the essentials of human value, dignity, and solidarity. The New Testament makes clear that God sometimes uses "the foolish things of the world to shame the wise, and . . . the weak things of the world to shame the things which are strong."[26] The meaning of life cannot exhaustively be described in terms of strength, independence, autonomy, physical and/or mental potentials, or quality of life. The presence of handicaps may put questions about the meaning of life in their proper context, i.e., relieved from superfluous additions, and leads human beings to ask what it is that *really* matters in a human life. This brings us to a view of man.

5.6. View of Man

A Christian view of man is characterized by the elements of rationality, self-determination (or autonomy), and responsibility. Humans are free to develop and use their capacities and are called to consent to their responsibilities. The quest for respect for human autonomy does have theological warrants. One of the merits of protestantism — in the form of Luther's "priesthood of all believers" — is its stress on the responsibility of every individual human being. Not without reason, humanism and protestantism grew up side by side. In later centuries, their ways parted and secular humanism disconnected the idea of autonomy from the notion of responsibility. Health care ethics enter the third millennium with a concept of autonomy which has become the foremost parameter for evaluating the quality and meaning of human life.

From a Christian perspective, autonomy has long-standing credentials. Humans are created in the image of God and one of its implications is the capacity to act as responsible stewards, to outline their own goals in accordance with the divine purposes, and to pursue these with all their capacities. This autonomy, however, is part of a larger conception of what it means to be human. In almost every respect, human beings are dependent upon conditions beyond their own power. These conditions make not only life and happiness possible, they also put limits to them. Just as life and individual human existence are a gift that no one has ever asked for, death will inevitably put an end to all human pursuing and boasting. Though the range of human action and influence has increased, human beings cannot alter their final fate. "In living and dying," as the Heidelberg Catechism says, "my only consolation is that I am . . . property of Jesus Christ." Man's freedom is therefore, in the words of Merleau Ponty, a "situated freedom." James M. Gustafson contends that " . . . [i]n most circumstances we are 'more acted upon than acting'."[27] This dependence pertains both to our factual possibilities to act, and to our volitional freedom to want, will, and intend. Gustafson therefore argues that "the radical transcendental freedom claimed for human beings in existentialist theologies does not pass the tests of well-established scientific views of 'human nature.'"[28]

From a Christian perspective, thinking of humans exclusively as autonomous agents not only flies in the face of factual circumstances, i.e., it is not only deceptive, but it is also undesirable. Part of a Biblical view of man is the assumption that full humanity implies the capacity to trust others, to "let go", to comply to decisions made by others, to be moulded by the company of fellow human beings, in short: to accept the conditions of dependency.

The more serious a mental retardation is, the more someone has to rely on the care of others. We may say that people with mental retardation reflect the aspect of dependence more than people with full mental capacities. They remind us of aspects of human existence which are common to all, but which are forgotten, repressed, or trivialized by many.

6. CONCLUSIONS

From a Christian perspective, there is no reason to downplay the severity of mental retardation. It is a form of non-moral evil — or, in other words, a tragedy — in creation which, other things being equal, should be prevented. At the same time, there is no reason to question the meaning of life of people with mental retardation. When it comes to meaning and dignity, people with, and people without mental retardation are in the same position, namely a vulnerable position. The Bible bases respect for human beings not on any of their singular properties, but on their being-created, on their being-redeemed and on their membership of the human community. On top of this, the prospect of a final restoration of all things is of paramount importance. Handicaps do not have the last word. The last word is that suffering, diseases and handicaps will be removed and this empowers people to keep up hope in situations where experiences of meaning are missing.

"Meaning" is an action-guiding concept. This forms the link between meaning of life and meaning of care on the one hand, and quality of care on the other hand.

NOTES

1 Cf. V. Brümmer, *Theology and Philosophical Inquiry: An Introduction*. London: MacMillan, 1981: "To ascribe meaning to something we might . . . use gerundive predicates that say more precisely what pro-attitude or con-attitude is appropriate to something", p. 122.
2 *Ibid.*, p. 121.
3 This can be compared to John Rawls' *Hypothetical Deductive Method* (HDM), which he uses for setting up a theory of political ethics. See J. Rawls, *A Theory of Justice*. Oxford: Oxford University Press, 1988.
4 For the same reason, it seems much harder to understand the "meaning of meaning" in cultures whose language we have not yet deciphered.
5 The Bible, Revelation 7:17, 21:4, *New American Standard Bible*.
6 Cf. Th.A. Boer, *Theological Ethics after Gustafson: A Critical Analysis of the Normative Structure of James M. Gustafson's Theocentric Ethics*. Kampen: Kok Publishers, 1997, pp. 287ff.
7 The British theologian Oliver O'Donovan describes the work of Christ, especially the resurrection from the dead, as *vindication of creation*. O. O'Donovan, *Resurrection and Moral Order: An Outline for Evangelical Ethics*. Grand Rapids: Eerdmans, 1986.
8 Matthew 5:3. Against this interpretation, it is argued, there is a parallel text in Luke 6:20, which only refers to "you who are poor." In order to harmonize the two texts, the "poor in spirit" in Matthew could be understood as "poor to the bone", "poor into their very existence". This last interpretation seems a bit far-fetched and it excludes the possibility that Jesus actually said both things.
9 In contrast to some voices within the New Age-movement, Christianity does not believe that mental retardation is the result of something equal to a deliberate choice of someone in a previous life.
10 Genesis 1:31 and Revelation 21:4-5, respectively.
11 The problem how to relate a good and powerful God to the presence of evil in creation, has traditionally been referred to as the *theodicy*. See, e.g., U. Görman, *A Good God? A Logical and Semantical Analysis of the Problem of Evil*. Lund, Sweden: Verbum, 1977.
12 Romans 8:28.
13 Leviticus 21:17-21, 22.
14 Leviticus 14 and 15:2ff., respectively. *Cf.* Leviticus 22:23.
15 In the service of sacrifice, it was not allowed to sacrifice animals with a defect, such as lameness or blindness (Deuteronomy 15:21). God's holiness and perfection cannot be represented by animals with defects. There is no reason, however, to assume a parallel here between animals and humans.
16 Jeremiah 31:8.
17 Matthew 5:3.
18 This discussion will be continued in other contributions in this book. See especially Chapters 6, 7, and 8.
19 Many non-moral forms of evil ("things happening to us") may be caused by moral negligence ("things done morally wrong"). For example, being exposed to nuclear radiation during early pregnancy may cause handicaps for the fetus. For the parents and the future child, this is a *tragedy*, caused by a *moral* wrongdoing by those who are responsible for the radio-active contamination.
20 When a person has to choose between two evils, this is a tragedy; only the decision to do the biggest of the two evils can be called moral evil, as R.M. Hare argues convincingly. See R.M. Hare, *Moral Thinking: Its Method, Levels, and Point*. Oxford: Clarendon Press, 1981. We meet the distinction between moral and non-moral evil in the well-known book of H. Kushner, *When Bad Things Happen to Good People*. London: Pan Books, 1982. "Bad" in the title refers to non-moral

evil which may incur, whereas "good" refers to moral qualities in human actors.

21 In a prophetic context, for example, when prophets interpret certain historic events as a Divine judgment; and in a pastoral context, which is characterized by a full and unconditional trust and confidence between two or more people. The counsellor and the prophet who identify such a link, are close to the people who need help and will normally be in a position to offer practical or pastoral follow-up. Outside a pastoral or a prophetic context, identifying a link between a particular tragedy and a particular sin which might have caused the tragedy is not only difficult, but may also be utterly harmful.

22 John 9:2-3.

23 Leviticus 19:14.

24 Deuteronomy 27:18.

25 John 9:3.

26 The Apostle Paul in I Corinthians 1:27.

27 J.M. Gustafson, *Ethics from a Theocentric Perspective. Part One: Theology and Ethics*. Chicago: University of Chicago Press, 1981, p. 283.

28 *Ibid.*, p. 269.

HANS S. REINDERS

CHAPTER 5

MENTAL RETARDATION AND THE QUEST FOR MEANING

Philosophical Remarks on "the Meaning of Life" in Modern Society

1. INTRODUCTION

The other day I saw a theatre-play about the lives of people with mental retardation that contained the following scene. A man who appeared to be autistic was working on a piece of stone with the size and shape of a large pebble. He was sanding it with sandpaper. It seemed as if he was at work. A metronome that he had set into motion was ticking on the table before him. He was very much "into" his work, although the activity itself appeared quite useless. Whatever it was that he was doing, sanding a pebble with sandpaper did not get him anywhere. His movements appeared mechanical, his face showed no particular expression or emotion. His hand seemed merely to follow the motion of time. But then he started to talk. It turned out that he wasn't on a job. That was only how it looked from outside. "I want to get inside of this stone," he said, "but it won't let me." He squeezed the stone between his hands as if trying to crack it, but failed. Then he picked up a piece of timber and knocked almost politely on the stone and waited. He then knocked a little firmer. Still there was no reaction from the stone. He got irritated with it and hammered it with all the force that was in him. After a few seconds the tension of his muscle relaxed. "The stone says I will not be allowed to enter. I keep trying though. I must. I know that there are large rooms in there, large ballrooms where one can dance, and dinner halls with long tables." Then he fell silent. A moment later he picked up the sandpaper and started sanding his stone again. After a few minutes he stopped, put away the stone and his tools and sat gazing at the ticking metronome with blank eyes and his face without expression. Finally he started to write on his working table while speaking the words that he wrote: "In the beginning is the end and the end is in the beginning."

This scene came to my mind when I was thinking about what to say on the subject of mental retardation and the quest for meaning, and, particularly, *how* to say it. It occurred to me that the scene conveyed a multi-layered message about "meaning". In a way it seemed as if the man himself was reflected in the stone. He

Joop Stolk, Theo A. Boer & Ruth Seldenrijk (eds.). Meaningful Care, 65—82

was that stone, a "thing" with an interior, but one that somehow refuses to open and give itself. At least there was the suggestion of interiority, expressed by the image of the pebble as filled with a decorated space. So it seemed there was something like the "inner" man, a mental space, a "soul", if only one could get in touch with it.

At the same time, however, the man seemed to show us how people respond to the suggestion of self-contained interiority: they want to get inside. Self-contained interiority in humans, particularly the ones we care for, is just too enticing to resist the will to open it. Remembering what I had seen of programmes for teaching severely disabled people communicative skills, it occurred to me that, maybe, the man was showing us how it feels to be surrounded by people who approach you as if you were a stone that needs to be opened. Your "soul" is closed and the very attempt to unlock it, however well intended, is a continuing reminder of the fact that you are imprisoned.

And what about the metronome and the words that where spoken about time? Were they about the stone or about the man? Or were they perhaps about the people surrounding him? Did the ticking metronome symbolize the timeless existence of the stone, of the man, or of both? Or did it reflect how the failure of getting "in touch" with a person renders the existence of that person as existing beyond time, not evolving between past and future, without beginning or end? When seen from the outside, does not a human being whose interior world is closed evoke a sense of timelessness that makes every moment appear to be just another tick of the metronome?

In this paper I will try to think about the quest for meaning in connection with mental retardation, particularly profound mental retardation. I will attempt to show that the quest for meaning as it is understood in modern society is, in a way, threatening our ability to respond to the lives of these people. The reason has everything to do with the connections between meaning, interiority and time. Many of our contemporaries seem to believe that the meaning of their lives is something of their own making. It is neither received nor discovered as being "out there", i.e. it is not inherent to external reality, but produced by their own reflection. In other words, the prevailing notion appears to be that, somehow, "interiority" is the source of meaning, beyond which there is no other source. This contemporary view of meaning is characterized by activist notions such as "giving", "constructing" and "inventing", which indicate the displacement of previous notions such as "receiving", "finding" and "discovering". At the same time, however, the modern quest for meaning tends to become totalitarian. It makes the meaning of all our activities dependent on "the big picture" to the effect that unless we can grasp the meaning of the whole of reality, we cannot be sure about the meaning of anything in particular.

In my account of this modern view, I will first try to explain the semantic shift noted above in some detail, including some of the key notions it involves. Then I will look in some detail at the philosophical background of the particular conception of meaning in modern times. The discussion will be largely theoretical, but it aims at showing the practical implications for our appreciation of people who are *incapable* of giving meaning to their lives because they lack an interior world, i.e. people with profound mental retardation. They in particular may appear to the outsider as ensouled, but closed "stones". Although these people will not appear in my argument until the very last stage, I hope it will become clear by then that I had them in mind all along the way.

With regard to people with profound mental retardation, one is occasionally confronted by sceptical views about the meaning of their lives. For example, when it is said that the lives of such human beings are pointless because they exist merely as "vegetables". I will argue that this sceptical view stands in the way of our ability to share our lives with such people. The claim of the sceptic is, basically, that given the absence of reflective experience, the lives of people with profound mental retardation cannot have meaning, because their lives cannot be meaningful to themselves. This is the claim I intend to challenge. However, my argument will not try to refute this claim by showing a way in which the profoundly disabled *can* be said to have meaningful lives even if their lives cannot be meaningful to themselves. Instead, I will attempt to undermine the quest for meaning that is implied in the sceptical view, both with regard to the conception of meaning that it presupposes and with regard to the claim that this meaning is constituted by an operation of the mind. It is this modern quest for meaning that alienates us from people who lack the capacities of the self, that is, the capacities of reason and free will.

In contrast, my suggestion will be that people will have no idea of what it means to share one's life with a person with mental retardation and to care for her unless they are actually engaged in doing it. It has been reported that parents of children with severe handicaps sometimes experience their lives as a rewarding journey, but only after they came to understand that nothing in their lives would ever change unless they opened themselves to the possibility that their child had something to give.[1] This does not only suggest that there is an element of receptivity constituting the meaning they found in parenting their disabled children. It also suggests that, in an important sense, the modern quest for meaning as the product of reflective activity is frustrating our ability to find meaning in particular kinds of activities, such as the activity of caring. I will argue that, unless we see the importance of these points, we are most likely to misunderstand what these parents are saying. If there is anything threatening to the future of disabled people in our society, it is the notion that we have to give meaning to our lives. But it will take us quite a while to reach this conclusion by means of philosophical analysis.

2. SOME CONCEPTUAL CLARIFICATIONS

Let me begin with the semantic shift between the two opposing sets of notions that were introduced above: "receiving", "finding" and "discovering" versus "giving", "constructing" and "inventing". Clearly, we cannot make too strong a distinction between these two sets, otherwise it must logically collapse. Even if "meaning" is a matter of receiving, we still need someone who is "doing" the receiving. The reverse is also true: even if meaning is a product, something that is made, we still need something it can be made of. We could not invent meaning from scratch even if we tried. The philosophical issue does not seem to lie in an "either—or".[2]

To identify the philosophical issue let me attempt a clarification of the concept of meaning that occurs in notions such as, for example, the meaning of life. What does it entail? There are many ways in which things can have meaning, but we may start by distinguishing between objects and projects on the one hand and words and phrases on the other. There are some poems that mean a lot to me, but were I invited to explain what that meaning is, I would not start with talking about the meanings of separate words and phrases. So, the meaning that these poems have for me cannot be reduced to the level of semantics. Let us distinguish therefore between "semantic" meaning and "existential" meaning. To say that a given object is meaningful to us existentially, whether it is a person, a thing, or an experience of something, is to express that we have a stake in that object. It is to ascribe prescriptive properties to that object.[3] To say that opera means a lot to me is to express a particular "pro"-attitude, a sensibility that I have for this particular form of art. "Meaning", in other words, is connected with value. In ordinary life, many "objects" have meaning in this *axiological* sense. Family dinner has a special meaning in many homes, because it is the only hour that the members of families meet together. To be absent one needs an excuse or at least an explanation. Our lives are filled with many such everyday experiences that are meaningful to us.

But even if there are these many meaningful experiences in their daily lives, people nevertheless can simultaneously experience a kind of emptiness, a void, a lack of direction. On the whole, the meaning of their lives escapes them. In most cases this is only a temporary experience that occurs occasionally, but not constantly. Whenever it does occur, however, the meaning of daily experiences tends to become illusive. The explanation for this possibility is given with a further characteristic of "meaning". Things appear to have meaning because they are embedded in larger structures. The family dinner has its specific meaning because of a complex pattern of expectations, values and institutional variables in family life, such as school and work — a pattern that informs our daily affairs. On this view, "meaning" is not attached to isolated things but is conferred upon objects by the larger context within which they have their proper place or function.[4] Consequently, it seems to be the case that whether or not our daily experiences have meaning is dependent on whether the larger context — "the big picture" — within which we have these daily experiences have meaning. And reversely, if the meaning of the larger context crumbles, the meaning of particular things tends to erode. The "big picture" operates as horizon against which our daily experiences fall into place. The possibility of experiencing meaning on the level of these experiences is seemingly dependent on this horizon. For example, going to church is meaningful to me in the context of being a member of a religious community; being a member of such a community is meaningful to me in the context of what my religion teaches me about my place and task in the world. Similar things can be said about any of our daily activities. Teaching a course in philosophy is meaningful to me because training students to think critically about important questions is meaningful and this, in turn, is meaningful because I believe that the world will be a safer place if people use their intellectual capacities in a self-critical way. In this connection "horizons", "contexts" and "levels" are designations that can refer to various things, not only intellectual frameworks but also social and cultural environments.[5]

This feature of *contextuality* explains why questions about meaning *in* our lives — the things we do, the people we meet — seem to have a tendency to slide back to the question of the meaning *of* our lives. The "big picture" which holds everything together may itself become unclear. Fortunately, questions about the meaning "of" are not constantly on our mind because the meaning "in" our lives does not constantly create problems. But occasionally such questions do arise. Occasionally the experience of embeddedness is missing, because the larger picture has been blurred or has collapsed. At such moments the meaning of life has turned into a problem. The question "what is the point of my life?" or "what is it that makes my life worth living?" makes people fall silent. They do not know what to say to that question. Consequently, they find themselves in doubt as to whether the things they value in their daily lives are as important as they usually think they are.

To summarize these conceptual clarifications so far, two characteristics of the concept of meaning have been identified. "Meaning" as in the notion of the meaning of life is understood as an *axiological* term. It reflects the fact that the object in question evokes a positive attitude. It is also *contextual* in that it is constituted by our experience of being embedded in larger structures and frameworks. What has not been clarified is the question in what sense "meaning" is also a *relational* term. One might suppose that beyond being contextual and axiological, "meaning" also refers to being involved in something that is external to oneself.[6] Being involved in this way expresses a relation with an object that, somehow, presents itself as meaningful to us.

However, the notion of an object presenting itself as meaningful seems to imply that meaning is something inherent to the object itself, which would imply that meaning is something to be discovered. In the modern view this idea of discovering meaning has become notoriously suspect, however, because it presupposes that meaning is part of the fabric of reality, of how things "really" are. Many of our contemporaries do not accept that meaning is *given* with reality *as such*. The notion of meaning as "given" is disturbing to the modern mind because it seems to contradict the belief in ontological freedom.[7] Human beings are self-projecting beings, it is believed, who have no fixed ends set before them. The ends that make our lives meaningful are chosen, not discovered. They are not given as inherent to some larger and ultimate, metaphysical structure, because such structures are also the result of our reflective activity.

This essentially "constructivist" view is characteristic for the modern view of humanity as being in control of its own destiny. Even when many of our contemporaries seem to have lost faith in the powers of humanity in this regard, that does not stop them from believing that at least individual human beings can choose who they want to be. Accordingly, on this view, my personal identity is a construct of which I myself am the constructor. Or, to switch to another metaphor, even if it is true that there are many actors on the stage of my life, I am nevertheless the director of the play. Thus the modern view denies that there is a reality "out there" that somehow shows itself as "meaningful". It makes external reality appear as a large screen on which our conceptions of meaning are projected, instead of its being a source wherein meaning can be discovered.

These remarks help us understand more clearly the peculiar aspect of these contemporary views on the meaning of life that are the focus of this paper. Characteristic for these views is that modern people consider themselves to be the "author" of their own lives. The meaning of life is what they make of it. Whatever meaning there is to be found, it is constituted by their self-conscious and reflective activity.

However, the language of construction introduced above can be misleading. Construction is the business of engineers who build whatever it is they make — tools, machines, tunnels, and bridges — literally from blueprints. But even engineers do not seem to have complete control over their constructive work, given the "resistance" of the material with which they work. Similarly, it appears to be impossible for human beings to shape their lives from blueprints because of the patterns of meanings in which they find their lives embedded. Particularly in contemporary society there is a multitude of such patterns available. What people do, apparently, is to inscribe their lives into these patterns and live accordingly. In shaping their lives, they do not construct their own model. Instead they choose from a possible stock of meanings that their culture has attached to various ways of living one's life.

Instead of the language of construction, the postmodern language of aesthetic creation seems to be more accurate, therefore. According to the postmodern view, personal identity is not constructed like an engineering project but is assembled according to the model of the *bricoleur*, to use Claude Lévi-Strauss' famous expression. The *bricoleur* is not a constructor but a collector. He does not work from a blueprint, but sorts out whatever materials he is able to find and puts his objects together from bits and pieces.[8] In the postmodern view of aesthetic creation we are shaping our lives in the manner of *bricolage*. We take apart, revise, weed out and put together, using bits and pieces from the variety of cultural ideas that our society has available. Some of these materials are inherited from previous generations, some are reassembled and some are invented.[9] On this view, living a meaningful life is an ongoing process of restyling. People have their own languages, expressing their own histories and the histories of their cultures and subcultures, without there being a core of fixed meanings that is universally shared. The identity of postmodern individuals is characterized by a high degree of plasticity: it develops on the crossroads of constantly shifting interferences of various spheres and modes of thinking. Individual identity, according to postmodern thinking, appears as a mixed bag of many possible meanings from which we as agents are free to choose which are more central and more peripheral. Postmodern identity is the identity of "nomadic subjects".[10] This means that people are not properly "at home" in a given world of meanings, but that they make use of available languages in order to arrive at new *metaphors* to express their own individuality. As Richard Rorty's "poetic" criticism of traditional philosophy indicates, they express their own meanings on the plane of language by stamping their mark on the languages available.[11] Consequently, in the postmodern view people live meaningful lives in the way of creative reassembling. A meaningful life is not a creation in the sense of a *creatio ex nihilo*, but a creation from available fragments of "meaning" that our culture has on offer. We cannot want just anything, but we can choose and use our cultural resources freely.

As this account shows, however, there is a strong continuity between modernism and postmodernism in this respect, notwithstanding the differences between constructing and assembling meaning. The continuity exists in their joint rejection of a given reality as the source of meaning.[12] In other words, in both views "meaning" is an expression of the self rather than an impression that the world makes upon the self. Or, better — since on the postmodernist view the self is not something "beyond" its own expressions — our lives are the product of reflective activity rendering coherent the fragments of "texts" that bring meaning to an otherwise empty world. Consequently, it appears that we have to dig deeper into the question about the *relational* aspect of "meaning" as understood in contemporary culture. A brief historical outline may help to understand what happened to this concept.

3. FROM THE SENSES TO "SENSE"[13]

The conception of meaning as described in the previous section is a fairly recent one in the sense that it presupposes a shift in philosophical orientation that occurred somewhere in the nineteenth century. In order to trace this shifting orientation we may briefly look at the words used in modern languages to indicate the phenomenon of "meaning". Both in the German and Dutch languages there is a connection between apprehension, experience and meaning that does not appear in the English language in the same way. The former languages establish a semantic connection between "meaning" and the senses. They speak about meaning as "Sinn" (Dutch: "zin"; French: "sens") which is semantically related to the operation of the senses, "die Sinnen".[14] There is in the English language also a semantic relation between "sense" and "the senses", of course, but the relations are not identical. In the German phrase "der Sinn des Lebens" (Dutch: "de zin van het leven"; French: "le sens de la vie"), the word "Sinn" does not correspond with "sense" but with "meaning".[15] The relation between "meaning" as "Sinn" on the one hand and the senses on the other is an illuminating one, because it suggests that at one point of time "Sinn" was attached to apprehension rather than reflection. That is, in contrast to the modern view that understands "finding meaning" as reflective activity, in earlier times it was understood as an activity of the senses. "Meaning" was a matter of perceiving and observing, which did not refer to mere sensuous experience, but implied an attitude of being attentive to and mindful about (like in the expression "observing the monastic rule"). Apprehending the exterior world required the mind to become actively involved, but its activity remained necessarily dependent on observation. What happened, probably under the influence of German idealism, was that this connection between observation and apprehension was dissolved and "Sinn" became the exclusive domain of the mind ("Geist"). This development was partly fuelled by the growing importance of language for the understanding of human experience. "Sinn" came to be understood as being properly at home in language as a structured totality. It referred to the world as comprehended by the human mind in language. Accordingly, the shift was from *"having a sense of"* as the result of the activity of perceiving and apprehending, towards *"making sense of"*, which reflects an increasing emphasis on propositional content. The operation of the senses as constitutive of the "sense" of the exterior world was replaced by the interior act of comprehension. Consequently, the ability of "seeing" the meaning of the world turned into a function of human interiority. It is the comprehension of the mind, not the apprehension of reality that constitutes meaning.

As indicated, connected with this shift in understanding the nature of "seeing" was a shift in understanding the object of apprehension. The shift towards the reflective activity of the mind presupposed the idea of the senses presenting bundles of sensuous experiences that as such made no sense, but that acquired their appropriate meaning in being coordinated by the mind. Consequently, there was a shift in emphasis not only from "exterior" to "interior", but also from "fragment" to "totality". The quest for meaning aspired to absoluteness. It was not so much concerned with the meaning of this or that object, but with "meaning" as such. Meaning changes from something *relational* into something *substantive*. Moreover, it acquires a dimension of ultimacy that it could not have as long as it was connected with perception and observation.

This shift explains why in the contemporary view "meaning" tends to be blended with "value" and "purpose". The exterior world is the world of "brute" facts that as such may or may not coincide with human objectives. Consequently, "meaning" goes beyond that which merely *is* and includes that which *can be* or *could have been*. In explaining notions such as "the meaning of life", or "the meaning of suffering", or "the meaning of love", we do not just refer to our actual experiences. Rather we interpret these experiences from the point of view of what they may be, or might have been if the world were in accordance with our intentions and purposes. Hence the fact that "meaning" has acquired a state of absoluteness that makes it equivalent to the whole of actual and potential reality. The result of this development has been that the opposition between "sense" and "non-sense" — which refers to truth and falsehood — has been replaced by the opposition between "meaning" and "meaningless". Meaningless, in this connection, is not so much equivalent to falsehood as to nothingness and emptiness. The German theologian Gerhard Sauter, to whom I owe these reflections, has stated the consequence of this absoluteness with respect to the quest for meaning as follows:

> To ask about meaning is no less than to ask about what is real. If we cannot find an answer to this question, there is no longer anything to which we can really cling. We have fallen out of the world and are groping in the void. The question of meaning has thus become a question of being or nonbeing.[16]

Accordingly, the quest for meaning has gained a prominence in contemporary culture that it did not have before. It is supposed to assist us in mastering the exigencies of human existence, notwithstanding the fact that it is doubtful whether that task can be fulfilled by any of our reflective activities. Anyhow, the disturbing consequence seems to be that the meaning of this or that action appears as doubtful as long as it cannot be subordinated to a larger structure. As Sauter puts this: in order to know how to live, we need to know what life means.[17] Our actions become doubtful to the extent that perceiving and observing the world as it is does not provide us with guidance as to what to do. Instead, observation and perception is reduced to interpretation. This is a fateful development, according to Sauter, because the distinction between the particular and the absolute tends to collapse.[18]

4. ORIENTATION AND JUSTIFICATION

To understand the relevance of these reflections for my concern in this paper we must finally look at what Sauter says about the distinction between orientation and justification with regard to meaning. It occurs to me that his reflections at this point provide us with penetrating insights to substantiate the claim that the quest for meaning is potentially destructive.

If human beings attend to observing the world, in the sense as explained, the question they face is how to respond adequately to what happens. By requiring a sense of the things that surround us, both in time and space, this question turns out to be a question of orientation. Human beings experience things as having a particular "Sinn" which elicits a particular response. The task they face is to respond at the right time in the right way. "Meaning" in this connection signifies a mediate determinacy of the things (objects, events, actions) that confront us. These objects, events, and actions occupy a given time or space that cannot be occupied by other things. In this determined world our lives evolve and we look for orientation as to how we should live. We look for the actual sense that the things in this world show us by being what they are. This determinacy allows us a "hold" on the world. It is not constituted by our reflection on what or how things are, let alone by our reflection on what might have been had other possibilities been realized.[19]

From the perspective of the modern quest for meaning, however, the fact that people have this sense of what things are and how they are, does not seem to satisfy them any longer. They are inclined to go beyond what is, and want to find meaning that includes what could have been. In Sauter's terminology: people are no longer satisfied by things that are "sinnhaft", they long for things that are "sinnvoll".[20] Whether objects, events, or actions are experienced as meaningful depends on the larger scheme of things in which they participate. "Sinnvoll" as "meaningful" are those things that have their meaning "fulfilled" in the sense of being ultimately meaningful.

This is a crucial point, because it shows that for things to be meaningful in the modern sense they have to be justified in the context of all possible alternatives. In the end, there are no objects, events, or actions that are meaningful *per se*. Everything that is depends for its meaning on "the big picture". Consequently, orientation has been replaced by justification. What does not fit, should not be.

> It is no longer enough to see that in specific actions and experiences the opposing possibility is excluded. It seems that we can remain aware of it against the background of what takes place and is done, and more than that, that we have to understand what takes place in terms of the fact that we know it to be set in a nexus that contains everything that is possible. Only thus do we seem to have the full world of the possible, and only in relation to it can we justify this or

> that actual experience or action. From this point onward we no longer need to say merely what happened (content); we have to understand why it happened (purpose).[21]

The problem is, of course, that it is not given to human beings — for reasons of their finitude and contingency — to have a clear and reliable grasp of ultimate reality. The necessity of knowing the meaning of everything in order to determine the meaning of anything is just too much for finite beings to aspire to. Sauter's criticism is not that the question is illegitimate — there are plenty of senseless events and actions in the world — but that any attempt to answer it must be illegitimate.[22] Human beings cannot conceptualize and theorize about ultimate reality other than from within their own limited experience and understanding because they are finite creatures. Consequently, every interpretation of "the big picture" necessarily elevates a particular object to the status of explaining and justifying the whole of reality. Well-known candidates for this status are, of course, "history", "religion", "power", or "labour".

This is far from an innocent enterprise, however. Justification of particular things in the context of a view of the whole of reality requires judgment, which implies inclusion as well as exclusion. Since any interpretation of the whole of reality is necessarily the product of reflective activity, this means that human activity is no longer receptive, but constitutive of ultimate meaning. The consequences of this "copernican" shift are far from harmless. As Sauter makes the point:

> The reconstruction of the world from the bottom up . . . finds out [better: "decides" H.R.] what may be called meaningful and what seems to be meaningless because it has no importance and is hard to comprehend. Explanations of basic actions no longer view it as enough to show what things are included as meaningful in a nexus of authoritative interpretations within a culture, religion, or society, as distinct from many other things that were regarded as meaningful by other cultures and in other times. The nexus of meaning of the world as such is now the basis by which to say whether an action has to be called meaningful. The point is not that always and without exception reality depends on the human positing of meaning. The point is that what is meaningful decides what will emerge as significant and it is humans who have a normative part in this. Not given meaning but the giving of meaning is what counts.[23]

Given human finitude and the contingency of the world from within which human beings reflect upon its meaning, the tendency towards making the meaning of life dependent upon the meaning of the whole of reality cannot but result in illusion. However, this is not merely tragic, but it is destructive because — as Sauter puts it — in setting the standard for what is ultimately meaningful, the human beings are forgetting their contingency and finitude. This manipulation is what makes the modern quest for meaning a dangerous enterprise.[24]

5. "MEANING" AS A BYPRODUCT OF HUMAN ACTIVITY

It occurs to me that Sauter's reflections reveal an important truth about the contemporary conception of "meaning". If his explanation of the modern quest for meaning is correct — as I think it is — it necessarily follows that it must end in failure. Since any interpretation of ultimate reality as the horizon of being cannot but reflect the mind as located in time and space, it is intrinsically limited and therefore cannot be what it purports to be. Time changes, people change — as do their experiences — so that their attempts to transcend the contingencies of the world must itself remain contingent. Consequently, the truth of the matter seems to be that whenever we find ourselves asking questions about the meaning of our lives, we cannot attempt to fill the void by our own reflective activity without self-deception.

There is, however, a different way of thinking about "meaning" that is much less demanding and more rewarding at the same time. "Giving meaning" as an intentional, reflective activity does not work because meaning is essentially a "by-product".[25] In other words: it is a gift in the sense that it cannot be produced deliberately but has to be received. To understand what this means, I suggest we compare meaninglessness with another experience that most people want to avoid, which is sleeplessness. Meaninglessness is, in a sense, like sleeplessness: the harder one tries to overcome it, the more manifest it becomes. Reflecting on sleeplessness, our mind gets in the way of falling asleep with the most likely outcome that we are even more awake than before. Something similar is true of meaning. The act of finding it is an unreflective one.[26]

To explain, let me focus once more upon the opposition between "giving" versus "receiving" meaning. The question is: why should the meaning of my life be subject to "receiving" or "discovering" rather than "giving"? Why should it be mistaken to think, for example, that I give meaning to my life by devoting it to the art of music, supposing that this is what I care about most? The answer must be that this way of putting the question makes the very act of giving meaning self-contradictory. If the art of music is what I care about most, this is not because I chose it for that purpose. I could never choose a life devoted to music or anything else as a way of giving meaning to my life. Meaning cannot be extracted from objects that our will deliberately presents to itself as options among which we can choose. If meaning is not found *in* what we do — singing, reading poetry, gambling, saying our prayers, playing football — we will not find it by deliberately choosing to do these things either. Music fascinates me, captures my imagination, kindles my passion — these are all experiences that happen to me rather than experiences that I *make* happen. Meaning is not something that we can make or produce, because it cannot be the object of deliberate intention. I cannot deliberately choose to find meaning in my life by devoting it to the art of music, because I cannot deliberately choose to be fascinated or excited or to become passionate about such a life. I cannot even choose to see the point of such a life, if there is one. To think that I can produce meaning by making music the cause of my life is to put the cart before the horse. Finding meaning as activity is a way of responding to what has already been found. Something "discloses", "presents", "reveals" or "shows" itself to us as meaningful. These terms suggest that the quest for meaning will fail if the objects examined are approached as the "raw material" of an empty world that carries no meaning in itself. This was, of course, one of Sauter's main points. "Meaning" demands that we open ourselves to being engaged by the world as it presents itself, that we direct our attention to that which appears as "sinnhaft".

This aspect of disclosure also explains why we are vulnerable in these kinds of engagements. In order to find meaning we have to open up and allow ourselves to be moved, to be excited, to be thrilled. The experience of meaning is therefore characterized by vulnerability.[27] "Meaning found" can wither away and disappear, thus becoming "meaning lost". That is why we cannot find meaning unless we are prepared to be hurt, to be disappointed and disillusioned. The vulnerability of meaning has as its counterpart that we cannot avoid exposing ourselves to the possibility of suffering. We cannot avoid, that is, facing our own vulnerability in the quest for meaning.

Where does this alternative account leave us with regard to the question about "meaning" as a *relational* term? It seems to me that the answer is something like the following. In being attracted to a life devoted to music, I can choose to "answer the call", but I can also refuse to answer it. In either case the "call" precedes the response, but it is only with the response that my activity comes into play. The possibility of "finding", in this example, is dependent on being involved in the practice of loving music. Such practices produce what Macintyre has called "internal goods".[28] These are goods that cannot be obtained other than by engaging in a specific activity and submitting oneself to the standards of excellence that govern it. To love music — and to do it well — requires skills that must be learned. The better one learns them, the more rewarding one's engagement in a given practice becomes. Thus practice mediates the possibility of being attracted by whatever it is that attracts. In other words: being attracted, excited, captured, moved — all of these notions signify "meaning found" in the experience of being engaged in a specific practice. Acting upon the standards of this practice signifies the other side, that is, "meaning found" as a response. My desire to achieve a particular goal is already a response to the attraction by the internal object of that goal, which impresses me and in which I want to take part in one way or another. Reflective activity is preceded by receptivity for what it is in the exterior world that appeals to our imagination. Without doubt, something like "finding meaning" as reflective apprehension must occur in the act of "finding", but it is properly understood as an act responding to what is perceived and observed as meaningful.

6. CARING FOR PEOPLE WITH MENTAL RETARDATION AND THE QUEST FOR MEANING

Given the modern view of "meaning" as being constituted by reflective activity it is not surprising that the lives of profoundly retarded persons appear to be meaningless in the eyes of those who are committed to this view. Consequently, it is also not surprising that sharing one's life with such a person must necessarily appear as a burdensome life that is tainted by a deficit of meaning. How could taking care of a human being whose life can have no meaning for itself not affect the meaning of that activity?

With regard to this kind of skepticism I want to make four comments, drawing upon the foregoing analysis. The first point is that to be capable of experiencing meaning in a life shared with a retarded person one has to care about that person. Without being personally involved, very little meaning can be found. Being engaged in their lives is where it all begins. Whatever meaning can be found will only be found in the context of the practice of caring. Suppose I am a friend of Jerry's who is a profoundly retarded young man with the "mental age" of a toddler. To say that Jerry means a lot to me is to say that there is something that attracts me not only to Jerry but also to his wellbeing. I could not leave him unhappy and remain equanimous about it. I would lose something. Furthermore, what I experience in caring about him, is not under my control. I cannot manipulate it. Taking Jerry out to the park, for example, is a meaningful activity because I know that he loves the sound of birds. I cannot make the sound of birds attractive to him nor can I make taking him out to the park meaningful to me. As explained before, meaning is essentially a "by-product". To find it we have to be engaged in doing something else and then receive it as an unsolicited gift. I already referred to the analogy with intending to fall asleep, but there many other examples of meaningful experiencing that cannot be the object of wilful, intentional activity. Reporters of soccer games occasionally observe that a particular player is not "in the game", or that a team is "playing against themselves". Being "in the game" means losing oneself in it. "Playing against oneself" means trying so hard to play well that one's intention gets in the way of succeeding. Experiencing meaning seems to have a similar structure. To find meaning we have to be "carried away" in the sense of being "outside" ourselves and engaged "in" the object. Only to the extent that one is capable of this kind of attentiveness and of losing oneself in an activity does the experience of fulfilment come, precisely because one's attention is not directed to that experience itself. The skeptical view, in contrast, is a view that betrays the perspective of the outsider. The outsider is not involved. Often she does not want to become involved because she takes to be consumed by disappointment and disillusion to be a waste of energy. In other words, the sceptical outsider is motivated by the desire to avoid vulnerability.

The reports of the parents portrayed in Kathryn Scorgie's study about what makes parenting a child with mental retardation a success, prove this point.[29] Parenting a retarded child transformed their views of life as well as of themselves, but these transformations only occurred after a moment of surrender in which they had no choice but to accept that their lives would never be what they originally planned them to be. Obviously, *if* we regard our children as a means to our own fulfilment, the presence of a child with mental retardation is going to cause a great deal of stress and frustration. Not only because the presence of such a child reduces our capacity to control our lives but also because we are committed to a conception of a meaningful life that is inevitably going to make our retarded child look like a failure. According to Scorgie's study, one of the things the parents had to learn is to define meaning in terms that are very different from what these notions mean in contemporary culture. The quality of their lives was more a matter of personal growth in respect of their character than in respect of status and success. One parent characterised this shift, as changing from a perspective that was goal-oriented to one that has an "attributional emphasis".[30] Meaning and success are related to *how* lives are lived rather than to the states of affairs they produce. Were "meaning" to depend on the extent to which parents succeeded in realising their original plan of life, their days would have been filled with negative coping, which is what remains once one cannot do what one really wants to do. However strong and self-confident these parents may appear, their strength and self-confidence have been gained only on the condition of accepting vulnerability and the loss of self.

The second point concerns the fact that "finding meaning" in this connection has very little to do, if anything, with the contemporary role model of the "achiever". Nor has it much to do with "feeling good about yourself because of what you do for others." From the point of view of these contemporary role models, the lives of people like my friend Jerry cannot appear as anything but a burden that frustrates their parents' goals. Consequently, the lives of those who care for such people look anything but "great" of "attractive" from the point of view of the self-gratifying confidence of the successful achiever. What can one possibly get out of one's life by caring for someone who does not even know he exists? The sceptical outsider who wants this question answered before deciding to become involved, will only see a life captivated by natural necessity. The difficult task of parenting a retarded child nullifies the options to lead an interesting, eventful life. It is time and energy consuming without many returns. Obviously the sceptical outsider will not deny people like Jerry's parents the "option" of caring for this boy if that is what they prefer, but that is as far as the spectator's appreciation of the lives of people like Jerry goes. In regarding "meaning" as the intended object of reflective activity rather than as a by-product of activities that I am engaged in for the sake of these activities themselves, I am myself in the way of experiencing anything as meaningful. In terms of the example: as long as the question what caring for someone like Jerry will mean to me must provide me with a reason to become engaged, I will hold back rather than give myself. I will block myself from the experience of whatever it is that can be found in spending my time with him. Whatever meaning is found, it will not be found unless I am motivated by different intentions than the intention of doing something meaningful.

My third comment is closely connected with this. The sceptical outsider may want to respond by saying that my analysis does not provide any specifically *moral* argument with regard to the issue of experiencing meaning in sharing one's life with someone with mental retardation. Apparently, I have tried in this paper to circumvent the moral point of sceptical view, which is that particularly the lives of profoundly retarded human beings are pointless to the extent that they themselves lack consciousness of their own existence. To argue against this view that it stands in the way of our ability to care for these people and share our lives with them is in no way to provide a *moral* reason why we should be willing to care for them in the first place. Arguing that this reason cannot be found outside of the activity itself is not only unsatisfactory on intellectual grounds, the sceptic might say, it is also wanting from an ethical point of view. Surely people can be morally mistaken in finding meaning as a by-product of an activity that is itself morally reprehensible. For example, members of oppressive religious sects may find meaning in their activity, but this would not by itself make their activity morally acceptable. Consequently, it seems that I cannot decline to refute the sceptical view and argue that the lives of the profoundly retarded *are* meaningful in themselves without making the decision to become engaged in their lives morally arbitrary.

There is a simple and a more complex response to this objection. The simple response is to say that becoming engaged in their lives is a necessary but not a sufficient condition for the possibility of finding a moral reason to care for the profoundly retarded. After all, that *is* what I have been saying against the sceptical view. The indirect strategy of the argument has been to show that the sceptical view depends on questionable intellectualist and constructivist assumptions about meaning that undermine our ability to give ourselves to certain practices of caring. The meaning that can be found in the experience of caring for a profoundly retarded person does not depend at all on whether living her life as it is, is meaningful to that person herself. Nor does it depend on whether the activity of caring for that person is meaningful to her. Instead meaning can be found in realizing valuable things for that person in a non-subjective sense. It exists in realizing the good of decent clothing, of providing opportunity, of being friends, of healing wounds, of comforting in times of sorrow, of enjoying a walk together, etc. It is only when one believes that the value of these goods disappears when they are not integrated and superseded by a conception that the person herself holds on her life as a whole — "the big picture" —, that the sceptical view succeeds. But this is the belief that I have argued to be mistaken, following Sauter's masterful distinction between "sinnhaft" and "sinvoll". The sceptical view depends on a "totalitarian" conception of meaning that annihilates the objective value that practices of caring have in them because of the goods they create.

With this "simple" response I have also indicated how the more complex response might run. If people can be mistaken about the meaning they find as by-product of their activity, their mistake must be that, contrary to what they believe, their activity as such does not create valuable things. People can be misguided in the nature of the goods they pursue, even though they can experience the pursuit itself as meaningful. In other words, my argument against the sceptical view presupposes an account of objective goods that provides us with a standard for moral evaluation. It is outside the scope of the present analysis to try and present such an account, of course. But I suggest that the practices of caring for other people create the kind of goods indicated above by way of example: providing food and clothing, making friends, offering comfort and companionship, and so on. Moreover, I suggest that if the activity of caring for others is to be performed well, it must be connected with caring about them.

The last point regards the question of whether the lives of profoundly retarded people can be meaningful to themselves. If the argument for meaning as a by-product succeeds, nothing depends upon answering it, on the contrary. As a matter of fact, the question of what the lives of such people mean to themselves is a potentially threatening one. The idea that "the meaning of life" is what individuals make of it has serious implications for human beings to which the notion of agency does not apply. It is this very ideal that makes their lives appear to be deficient. Where there is no agent, there must be a deficit of meaning. Where a deficit of meaning exists, human existence must appear as the cause of suffering. If it is a cause of suffering, the question of why these people are kept alive becomes hard to avoid indeed. Not only is it hard to avoid, it also appears to have a definite answer. The centrality of agency and all that it stands for — "choice", "decision", "freedom", "self-determination" and so on — is the default position of contemporary culture. It makes us blind to other dimensions of our existence, such as our lack of control, our vulnerability and our dependence on other people. By the same token, accepting retarded people as human beings in their own right, without expecting them to meet contemporary standards of success, becomes a difficult task indeed. In our days the question as to whether profoundly retarded lives have meaning in themselves creates a vexing, almost paralysing problem. What I have been trying to do in this paper is to dislodge this problem — not by trying to solve it but by opening a different perspective that makes it look less important. Once the conceptual framework that generates the problem is displaced, there is no reason to think that the problem must be solved before one can meaningfully share one's life with someone like Jerry.

NOTES

1 K.I. Scorgie, *From Devastation to Transformation: Managing Life When a Child is Disabled* — Dissertation (Edmonton: University of Alberta), 1996.

2 This is the central question in W. Stoker, *Is The Quest for Meaning the Quest for God? The Religious Ascription of Meaning in Relation to the Secular Ascription of Meaning. A Theological Study*, tr. Lucy and Henry Jansen, Currents of Encounter, Vol. 11. Amsterdam/Atlanta: Rodopi, 1996. See particularly pp. 170-79 where Stoker opposes the philosophical positions that take both notions as representing alternative conceptions of meaning, respectively the "objectivist" (finding) and "subjectivist" (giving). He considers both positions to be false, because the subjective and objective aspects of meaning cannot be separated (p. 171).

3 V. Brümmer, *Theology and Philosophical Inquiry: An Introduction*. London: MacMillan, 1981, p. 121.

4 Stoker (1996) pp. 6-7.

5 An interesting question is how one should conceive of the connections between various levels and structures. Traditionally, theologians are the ones who think that religion — and therefore ultimately God — is the most encompassing "entity" for conferring meaning upon our lives. That is to say, in their view God is equivalent to "ultimate reality" (to borrow Paul Tillich's term) or to "the whole of reality" (as Wolfhart Pannenberg has it). Stoker's book is a theological attempt to take the rejection of this particular claim by secular thinkers seriously. The opposite (secular) position regards the outstanding feature of modern existence to be the fact that people construct their own images and hierarchies of heaven and earth. Consequently, in this view, being a fan of Amsterdam's famous soccer club *Ajax* can confer meaning upon one's daily experience just as any religion may do. The opposite theological position regards the modern quest for meaning to be grounded in forgetfulness about human finitude and contingency. This is the position held by Gerhard Sauter, whose argument we will consider later in this paper.

6 See R. Nozick, *Philosophical Explanations*. Oxford: Oxford University Press, 1981, p. 594.

7 The belief in ontological freedom — i.e. the belief that objects are not just instances of an essence that determines what they "really" are, with the result that their particular properties are merely "accidental" — does not stand on its own, but is on a par with other beliefs such as the belief that any statement about the essence of things cannot be separated from our conceptual schemes. I owe this point to Jan Bransen.

8 C. Lévi-Strauss, *The Savage Mind*. Chicago: University of Chicago Press, 1966, p. 17.

9 See J. Stout, *Ethics after Babel: The Languages of Morals and their Discontents*. Cambridge: James Clarke & Co, 1988, pp. 74f. It will be recalled that Lévi-Strauss uses the metaphor of *bricolage* in order to characterize the premodern mind that operates in a non-constructionist way.

10 Cf. R. Braidotti, *Nomadic Subjects: Embodiment and Sexual Difference in Contemporary Feminist Theory*. New York: Columbia University Press, 1995.

11 R. Rorty, *Contingency, Irony and Solidarity*. Cambridge: Cambridge University Press, 1989, pp. 3-22; pp. 23-43.

12 See Rorty (1989) pp. 39ff. where he explains the shift towards radical contingency in authors such as Nietzsche and Proust as the appreciation of the power of redescription, which is "the power of language to make new and different things possible and important — an appreciation which becomes possible only when one's aim becomes an expanding repertoire of alternative descriptions rather than The One Right Description. Such a shift in aim is possible only to the extent that both the world and the self have been de-divinized."

13 In this section and the following I am heavily depending on G. Sauter, *The Question of Meaning: A Theological and Philosophical Orientation*, trans. and ed. by Geoffrey W. Bromiley. Grand Rapids: Eerdmans 1995, particularly Chapters II and III. I should make explicit that Sauter's main interest is theological in that he intends to criticize the modern quest for meaning from a Christian point of view and, therefore, is rather suspicious of attempts to *resolve* the quest for meaning by suggesting "religion" as an answer. Although I will leave the question of whether his critique can be justified within a secular frame of reference, I do believe that it can be articulated in terms of human experience, that is, without using religious language.

14 Sauter refers to the German dictionary of the Grimm brothers to show that "Sinn" means an orientation of the mind, equivalent to the latin term "sensus". In earlier developments "Sinn" was connected with perception and observation, Sauter (1995) pp. 5-6.

15 The Shorter Oxford English Dictionary has for "sense" the faculty of perception, or the actual perception. Interestingly, the term "meaning" is used for intention and purpose, or having intention or purpose. As we will see, this difference matches precisely the distinction between two uses of "Sinn" that Sauter is after.

16 Sauter, *o.c.*, p. 11.

17 *Ibid.*, p. 13: "In short, meaning in the absolute is needed if we are to be able to live. This is what it now means to ask about meaning."

18 *Ibid.*, p. 17.

19 *Ibid.*, p. 23.

20 There is a significant connotation in both these terms that should not go unnoticed. "Sinnhaft" is something on which "Sinn" "haftet", that is, "is attached to" or, perhaps, "participates in". "Sinnvoll" on the other hand is something that is "voll" with "Sinn" in the sense of being "fulfilled" or "completed". "Sinnhaft" indicates appropriateness; "sinvoll" indicates plenitude.

21 *Ibid.*, p. 25.

22 It appears to me that at this point Stoker's interpretation of Sauter's position is mistaken. Stoker objects to Sauter's judgment that the modern quest for meaning is "demonic", because some answers may be such, but that does by itself not disqualify the question as illegitimate. However, this is very close to what Sauter argues in his reading of the book of the Ecclesiast when he says: "Es genügt zunächst zu sehen, dass Kohelet eine Unterscheidung getroffen hat, die Ihm nicht verbietet, nach Sinn zu fragen — die es ihm aber versagt, Sinn gewinnen zu wollen. Sinn würde er hervorbringen, indem er das, was ihm begegnet und was er tut, in den Zusammenhang einordnet, den er für sinnvoll hält" (*Was heisst nach Sinn Fragen?* München: Chr. Kaiser, 1982, p. 35). The English translation of this passage clearly misses the point. It reads: "It is enough for us to note that the author has made a distinction so that he may ask after meaning but not try to achieve it himself. He will arrive at meaning if he takes that which encounters him and that which he does and integrates them into the nexus that he views as meaningful" (Stoker 1996 p. 28). The point missed is the rejection of "mastering" the problem of meaning, which is what one does by subordinating all actions and events into one's conception of the ultimately meaningful. Given Sauter's claim that the modern quest for meaning strives towards absoluteness, he does not think that there can be *any* valid answer, given finitude and contingency, even though this by itself does not invalidate the question.

23 Sauter (1995) p. 39.

24 Here again I disagree with Stoker, who argues that Sauter fails to distinguish between, and therefore confuses, two different senses of "meaning". On the one hand there is the "metaphysical" sense — similar to what I called the "contextual" aspect — which says that meaning is dependent on ultimate reality, and on the other hand the "teleological-subjective" sense — similar to what I called

the "axiological" aspect. Stoker's objects to Sauter's claim that the quest for meaning results in manipulative answers, while this is only a characteristic of the second but not of the first aspect (Stoker, *o.c.*, pp. 196-197). It occurs to me that Sauter is right in suggesting that the act of comprehensive reflection constituting "Sinn" in the modern sense *is* manipulative because it necessarily strives towards coherence. In this connection his critique of sociology — particularly Luhmann — appears to be on the mark when he says that sociologists claim that "[I]t is by selecting from what is objectively meaningful in experience and action that we achieve a meaningful context for life" (Sauter, *o.c.*, pp. 42-3). Luhmann's notion of "Kontingenzbewältigung" clearly expresses this manipulative sense. It indicates that events, actions, and objects in themselves are meaningless but acquire meaning only in the context of a larger whole which to provide is the task of cultural formations and processes. In other words, the "metaphysical" and the "teleological-subjective" are different aspects, but not distinct conceptions of "Sinn". The former is logically implied in the latter insofar as the "teleological-subjective meaning" aims at the mastering of contingency by striving towards coherence.

25 This notion is explained in J. Elster, *Sour Grapes: Studies in the Subversion of Rationality*. Cambridge: Cambridge University Press, 1983, pp. 43-108.

26 See G.M. van Asperen, "Eén temidden van velen: zingeving en ethiek" ("One Among Many: The Quest for Meaning and Ethics"), in: G.A. van der Wal and F.L.C.M. Jacobs (eds.), *Vragen naar zin* (The Quest for Meaning). Baarn: Ambo, 1992, pp. 86-103. The author argues that "The demand for reflexivity in modern societies is incomparably more intense than in a traditional society, where there is an undisputed consensus about meaning and purpose. Whenever the (legitimate) demand for reflexivity is translated as a demand for total transparency, as the demand to give a rational foundation for that by which one is motivated, then this is asking too much" (p. 97, tr. by the present author).

27 Stoker, *o.c.*, p. 203.

28 A. MacIntyre, *After Virtue: A Study in Moral Theory*. Notre Dame: University of Notre Dame Press, 1981, pp. 175f.

29 See above note 1. Scorgie's study investigates the characteristics of parents who claim that the task of parenting a disabled child has brought them a rewarding life. The characteristics she found have to do with changed attitudes towards life, changed conceptions of themselves and of what it means to be succesful. They have been "transformed". Scorgie's claim is not that this is generally true of parents with disabled children, nor that parents who do not share this experience are bad parents, but only that the experience of living a rewarding life occurs and reflects a particular kind of rationality. On this rationality see Chapter 11, "The Transformation Experience" in my forthcoming book *The Future of the Disabled in Liberal Society* (Notre Dame University Press).

30 Scorgie (1996) pp. 151ff.

SECTION THREE

MEANING IN MEDICAL CARE

RUTH SELDENRIJK

CHAPTER 6

MEANING IN MEDICAL CARE FOR PEOPLE WITH MENTAL RETARDATION

Some Remarks from the Dutch Context

1. INTRODUCTION

Many of us are probably familiar with the concept of *Ciconia*, or the stork.[1] The Dutch used to tell their children, "the stork will be visiting soon"; a relevant piece of information, since storks delivered babies. The stork didn't always deliver babies as desired, however. Nor did babies always live. Even so, nobody ever thought twice about taking up the responsibility of caring for the newborn child. This care was considered meaningful, since this new human being was accepted as a member of the human race. In those days, having children was still considered a natural process.

A new life is delightful, sweet, and tender; just starting to bud and not yet fully grown — a marvel to those who are aware of how it is developing. For that reason, when announcing a pregnancy, we often refer to it joyously as "expecting" a baby. But the conception and dawn of new life is not always a case of pure joy; at times a shadow is cast over the joy and we are faced with heavy questions, including questions about the meaning of life.

Questions of this kind have become all the more poignant because modern medicine has changed. Instead of respecting human life, medicine shows increasing tendencies to relativize life. Human life is no longer categorically respected, and its protection has become more and more bound to certain conditions. Some events from the Dutch context will illustrate this. In 1971, the Royal Dutch Association of Medicine issued its directives concerning abortion. In 1981, abortion was made possible by law. In 1999, the Dutch government launched a law proposal which extended the criteria and which now allows abortion up to a pregnancy of 24 weeks, i.e., the beginning of the child's viability. In 1993, the Dutch parliament accepted a law which allows euthanasia under certain conditions. Since 1995, these conditions even include serious *psychological* suffering while the patient no longer has to be *terminally ill*. In a law proposal of 1999, the conditions were further extended. In all these cases, the autonomy of the individual person — the mother of a fetus, a patient

Joop Stolk, Theo A. Boer & Ruth Seldenrijk (eds.). Meaningful Care, 85—99

— increasingly dominates the doctor's decisions, and threatens to push notions about meaning to the margin.[2]

My contribution is the first of four. This chapter provides a general introduction to problems encountered in the field of neonatology (where choices for life and death seem unavoidable), from a Dutch angle. Chapter seven discusses the change in values in medical practice, especially related to genetic analysis and prenatal diagnosis. Chapter eight discusses some cases of very premature children. The last chapter of this section deals with the results of an empirical study about parent's views on medical care in relation to the prevention of handicaps.

2. NEW POSSIBILITIES

The attention of the paediatrician has been directed increasingly to the earliest moments of child development. Out of neonatology (the area of paediatrics that is concerned with the care of infants) springs perinatology (concerned with the time period surrounding the birth). Even prior to the birth, the paediatrician and gynaecologist discuss the health risks of the unborn child.

This past decade, great improvements have been made in obstetrics and neonatology. There are greater possibilities in medical technology and nursing, as seen in diagnostics (e.g., lab tests from one drop of blood, echography), interventions (pharmaceutical and surgical possibilities thanks to micro-technology), and health care (e.g., incubators). Due to these improvements, fetal and infant mortality rates have decreased from 35 per 100 in 1950 to 10 per 1000 in 1996 in the industrialized countries.[3] There are some notable differences in mortality rates (perinatal and newborn) in cultural minority groups. In the Netherlands, these differences are due to cultural adjustments rather than socio-economical status.[4]

Causes of pre- and perinatal defects and death include insufficient delivery of oxygen and nutrition to the newborn, prematurity, and genetic and congenital conditions. In the Netherlands, 7000-10,000 children are born per year with a genetic or congenital condition (4-6% of full-term infants). Newborns are especially at risk for asphyxia: a lack of oxygen during the birth process (2.9 - 9 cases per 1000 births).[5] The resulting risk for brain damage varies and is difficult to predict. For this reason, the asphyxiated neonate is always resuscitated; but at what point should this be stopped? More generally stated: should everything be done to keep the newborn alive? Should an intervention always be continued once it has been initiated?

For the neonatologist, the greatest causes for concern are very premature infants and infants with congenital conditions and handicaps.[6] Picture an incubator with an infant born three months premature, weighing less than 1000 grams (accounting for about 1% of the infants in the neonatal intensive care unit).[7] The organs of these infants are not completely developed yet. This vulnerable infant is therefore kept alive artificially by means of parenteral nutrition and mechanical respiration in combination with surfactant therapy. This phospholipid decreases the surface tension in the lungs by its presence in the mucous membranes of the alveoli, and aids greatly in preventing hyaline membrane disease, which used to be deadly. This infant receives cardiac support and intensive antibiotic therapy to prevent infection and is assessed and observed by means of a network of wires and tubes. A tangle of wires is connected to a series of monitors that measure pressures and other vital capacities. Functions the infant cannot maintain on its own, such as circulation and respiration, are substituted for mechanically. For example, certain newborns with acute respiratory difficulties temporarily receive ExtraCorporeal Membrane Oxygenation (ECMO). With this modern medical intervention, the infant's lung function is completely taken over mechanically for some time.

Until recently, these infants were doomed to die. Because of recent developments in neonatology, an increasing number of infants of greater prematurity can be saved from dying. Certain conditions that used to be considered untreatable have now become treatable. Because of improved health care and advanced treatment interventions, the risk for handicaps has decreased. As a result, these little ones have gained a more hopeful outlook on life. This leads to a feeling of power on the one hand, but on the other hand, no one has a strong grip on the situation anymore.

3. THE DOWNSIDE

There is another side to the picture. We now bear the responsibility for issues that we have never had to face before. There are some infants for whom the improvements described above do not make a difference. Specifically, one area that we can't seem to tackle is that of the central nervous system. Due to hypoxia or haemorrhage, these children often end up with some sort of brain damage. At times, the treatments these infants receive can lead to blindness. Other possible complications include pneumothorax (= air in pleural cavity between the chest wall and the lungs), pneumopericardium (= air in the sack surrounding the heart), patent ductus arteriosus (duct that stays open between the bend of the aorta and the pulmonary artery), as well as other complications. Despite the intensive care, some infants still end up dying. Others stay alive but, possibly a result of interventions, end up with serious disabilities.

These facts bring certain questions to mind. Is what we have accomplished truly progress? For instance, is it progress to be able to announce that several children of 22 weeks gestation have been saved, all of which are all completely blind? In 1983, the death rate of 27 week gestation premature infants was 43 percent, which has declined to 15 percent in 1997. The trend to keep increasingly premature infants alive continues. Before 26 weeks gestation, the problems of prematurity are much greater and the risk for handicaps, in particular visual, increases dramatically. Does the well-being of one patient measure up against the suffering of another patient brought on by the same intervention? In the latter case, was the intervention a service to the patient? If not, does the continuation of treatment and care still coincide with the ultimate purpose of medicine, which is to eliminate and alleviate suffering, and what exactly is necessary to accomplish this? Usually, we see in hindsight whether or not the decision to treat was the correct one. At that point, a more accurate diagnosis and intervention can be provided.

Presently, if the treatment and care given do not bring about improvements, we are faced with a new series of questions. These are provided in reports issued by the Royal Dutch Association of Medicine and the Dutch Association for Paediatrics.[8] The latter report contains a list of guidelines for the conversation between physicians and parents. It lists the following criteria for practical quality of life: a) *communication*: verbal as well as nonverbal communication is addressed. It pertains to psychological abilities and the ability to express these; b) *independence*: this concerns the results of an altered sensor-motor development, as far as possible in functional terms: mobility, independent sitting, self-care abilities, writing, ability to perform household and work duties, and creative abilities; c) *dependence on the medical circuit* (i.e., frequent hospitalizations, out of home placements, etc.) versus being able to live at home with minimal medical supports. The parents' ability to care for the child is also considered. d) *suffering:* pain and other forms of physical suffering play a large role with some conditions, but even other criteria are included when considered a burden to the patient. Also included are altered stool and urinary patterns, and the experience of being handicapped. e) *life expectancy:* in the case of severe suffering, a long life would be experienced as an extra burden, whereas on the other hand, the assurance that the child will in a short time die spontaneously could give room for simply waiting for nature to take its course. Both organizations suggest that, under certain conditions, humanitarian considerations justify the conclusion that an infant with profound multiple handicaps should be allowed to die. It is difficult for physicians to find the limits of their possibilities. The decision for death is made for two reasons. First of all, the expectation should be that "the hope for survival is unrealistic." This is based on more or less objective criteria in which a scoring system is used to create a prognostic statement. The second option is that the infant's life is predicted to be "unlivable" in the future, a term which does not take into account the value of life.

M.J.K. de Kleine *et al.*[9] performed a research study in four Dutch neonatal intensive care units. Of those children who had died in their intensive care unit, it appeared that of 31% (which is 5% of the children that were hospitalized), treatment was discontinued because it offered "no chance". For 19% of the expired children (3% of those hospitalized), the discontinued treatment offered no hope for a "livable life". In situations such as these, the question arises as to how the dying process should be facilitated.

Since the criterion of the "unlivable life" has a subjective character, we have reason for critical reflection on a number of issues, such as: how do we make decisions in ambiguous situations? What is a consistent way of managing different ideas? What are the ethical aspects of neonatology?[10] New possibilities cause more and more aspects of human life to be the object of choice, many of which used to be out of human control. With all the new possible options available, we have to realize that there is no moral choice without a moral price. The practical necessity of ethics is especially obvious in situations where people are subject to the right of the strongest!

4. MAKING CHOICES

Because of advances in the bio-medical sciences, we are faced with more and more choices[11], such as:

- whether or not to make use of the latest reproductive techniques,
- whether or not to be subjected to increasingly refined prenatal examinations,
- whether or not to maintain the pregnancy at the cost of the child when fetal deviations are present
- whether or not to provide care or intervention to a newborn with a profound handicap, etc.

Using the words of the Royal Dutch Association of Medicine — following an international trend —, we now talk of "seriously defective newborns". This type of language is not conducive to the bonding process of the newborn and the parent, which is so important — even when the parent needs to let go of the child.

The category, "seriously defective newborns" includes children with serious congenital anomalies and the high-risk population of largely premature infants that present with life-threatening conditions or handicaps. The concept, "newborns", defined by neonatology as the age range of 0-4 weeks, is often used for the broader range of 0-3 months (we will return to the question of whether and when an embryo is a person below). This is done because it is not easy to give an unfavorable prognosis with expected outcome of death in the midst of an acute situation; making a decision to end life is often not possible during the first month.

If desired, some risks and uncertainties can be eliminated before the birth by means of testing and consultation. The ultimate request would be one of complete certainty: the irrealistic and dubious demand to be guaranteed a healthy child. Symptoms visible at birth, such as with a newborn with Down's Syndrome, may be indicative of the chances for survival, but they usually do not provide sufficient information as to the level of mental retardation later in life. Moreover, physicians and nurses usually have inadequate experiential knowledge of what life is like with a mental retardation. The medical care of people with mental retardation has many specific aspects. This is related to the etiological diagnosis and the specific somatic and psychiatric comorbities (that appear along the way), the living and housing patterns, and the necessity to communicate with the family and/or care-givers. On the basis of practical experience and the increasing measure of reset in this area, a specialty area has been developing which may one day be acknowledged as such.[12]

C. van de Vate suspects that the more deontological ethos of parents as compared to the more consequentialist ethos of physicians could lead to miscommunication (*cf.* chapter nine).[13] Another cause for miscommunication may lie in structural problems, such as the lack of comfort with handicaps on the part of physicians, their ethos, and their lack of communication skills. On the other side of the spectrum, the lack of preparedness of the parents for what just hit them may contribute to communication problems. Working through these issues and coming to acceptance are processes that require time. In the meantime, the child with the handicap is at the receiving end of the miscommunication between physicians and parents, with the possible result that a decision to end the child's life is made wrongfully.[14] Therefore, with regard for the legitimacy of the life of this child, it is essential to do everything we can in order to have good communication. Bringing in other parents with personal experience (such as from parent associations) may help, since they can contribute by representing the concerns of the child.

Prospects for the life of the newborn with a profound handicap are associated with how society attributes normative meaning.[15] Societal developments are essential factors in the foundation of this normative meaning attribution. Three current developments that predominate in Western societies are individualization, judicialization, and economization.

The *individualization* sees human beings primarily as individuals, disconnected from social groups and institutional links. Individualization leads to a decreasing sense of community and solidarity. At the expense of other values, it emphasizes independence, autonomy, self-determination, emancipation, co-determination, and self-reliance. The paradox of human life is that in every area the person is a social being and at the same time strives for optimal self-development. Never before have people been as responsible for the management and direction of their own lives as in this present time. A handicap doesn't fit into this development, and is therefore usually reduced to an individual problem; the person has become this way due to some organic damage that has affected the quality of his existence.

A second development is the *judicialization* of society and health care. The Western mode of thinking focuses on rights and freedom. Even current thought-patterns regarding individualization contain a strong affinity for this model. It always concerns distanced relations between free and equal persons who are capable of will and action, and who are able to defend their own cause. Interpersonal relationships are seen in the perspective of (quasi-)contractual relations as a result of negotiations between equal parties. When applied to close, intimate relationships (life-partners, parents and children, friends, etc.), this leads to quite a distorted picture. Moral notions such as consideration, sympathy, loyalty, trust, love, and caring assume human bonds that are richer than the freedom- and justice model allows. There are signs that while our society increasingly values the *rights* of people, our sense of *duty* or obligation is fading more and more out of the picture. Recipients of health care tend to see themselves as consumers who are "in charge". This is reflected in their behaviour. As a result of increased concern for human autonomy, present-day conceptions of medical ethics have become strongly intertwined with the law. When the autonomous individual takes a central position, there is a strong temptation to formulate the wishes and concerns of the individual in terms of the rights (s)he possesses. Resultingly, a thought-process is created in which what is morally acceptable concurs with what is legally regulated and permitted. Since the substance of various ethical approaches can differ, there is a tendency to let the law provide for the forming of minimal consensus. Accordingly, involvement of a lawyer is increasingly common in the resolution of problems. The calculating citizen (a phenomenon of increasing individualization) translates his damaged rights into a claim for financial compensation. In the past 20 years, the number of lawyers in the Netherlands has increased fourfold.

Thirdly, due to society's *economization*, categories of people such as new graduates, the unemployed, the elderly, the sick, and the disabled all are affected by economic fluctuations. Rather than valuing them as they are, society tends to evaluate its citizens in terms of how much they contribute to society (a calculation of utility). Does it make sense to put out so much money for certain people if it does not lead to a general improvement in the quality of living? These relatively low-effective forms of medical treatment are characterized as "marginal medicine". This "marginal medicine", or "last chance medicine" is placed between ineffective and undesirable because of, among other reasons, economical considerations, or "because an earlier death can be in someone's best interest." Shouldn't we weigh the quality of life against economic costs? In debates as to which government policies in the field of health care are desirable, we see an increasing use of economic language. For instance, in the Netherlands, it has been calculated that it costs the Dutch government the equivalent of approximately 2 million US$ to provide for a man with Fragile X syndrome. With this mindset, one automatically starts to wonder for what other purposes we could be using that money.

Combining health care developments for premature and handicapped newborns with the growing list of wishes of society makes for a complex dance. It is the weak, non-economical, imperfect, defective, handicapped life that comes most under pressure. The economization and business-like nature of current living has led to a changed appreciation of lives. Science has given the vision of new life a different bend, bringing it down to a scientific process. It sounds paradoxical, but in our days the child is often considered to be a scarce product which is greatly valued; people go through great lengths to have one. On the other hand, the respect for the child seems to be lost. When health care developments are based on the wishes of society, processes like these seem unstoppable. As a result, societal and medical contexts create the risk that parents get a mixed-up and negative picture of the life of their newly born child.

Explicitly or implicitly we sometimes hear how "life can be worse than death". Natasja is the second child of a young family.[16] At birth, a large tumor-like protrusion is found in her lower back (meningomyelocele), and Natasja has neurological deficits in both of her legs. The neurosurgeon does not consider there to be an emergent need for surgical correction. Because it is suspected that Natasja has pain around the meningomyelocele, because she "has no prospect for a life worth living due to her defects," and because it is better not to let too much time pass during which the parents could bond with Natasja, she receives a calcium infusion the following day.[17] In a medical commentary on this case, neonatologist C. Versluys states that, considering the statement of the neurosurgeon, he would have foregone any palliative procedures with the possibility of future interventions such as surgery. He would also forego palliative procedures ultimately followed by life-ending actions if complications were to occur, but would choose instead to end her life puposefully unless a natural death caught up with him during the first weeks of life. "Considering my inner refusal to allow human suffering to take its "natural course" without exception, the only question that remains is: how do I provide the best possible death for this child? [. . .] I do not find this involuntary suffering (or a life that benefits no one) to be meaningful, or destined by an almighty God, but see it as a grievous crack in our existence, that begs to be healed. This doesn't mean that we cannot find meaning in dealing with suffering. [. . .] For Natasja, death is the best we have to offer. [. . .] In short: given the decision to forego surgery, my personal judgment is that I would be failing Natasja and her parents in choosing palliative interventions, while the purposeful ending of life in such a questionable case would be in line with my solidarity."[18]

When parents state that "life can be worse than death", they may be prevented from seeing the meaning of life of their child with mental retardation and prevents them from bonding with the child; thus, they tend to deliver their child over to die. This tendency is exacerbated if finances are taken into consideration in choosing whether to treat or not. A poor prognosis of the patient's situation naturally requires health care providers to do something about it; whether this provides reason to actively take the patient's life if no relief or treatment can be given, however, is not at all evident.

There is a growing conviction that our duty to protect a child does not start at conception but rather that it develops with the fetal stage of development. When is an embryo a person? In this age-long discussion, the start of human life is pushed further and further back. Some assume that it begins at conception (i.e., the last phase of fertilization), or 5-7 days later at the nidation, when the implantation of the conceptus in the uterine wall takes place (i.e., the first phase of pregnancy). Others contend that human life begins when the heart of the 7.5 mm long embryo beats on the 23rd day after conception, or when movements can be noted (between the seventh and tenth week). Yet others believe we should wait until the brain functions and reflex arcs have been established (about the twelfth week). Not only is the beginning of human life pushed back by doing this, the protective status of this life is pushed back as well. This also counts for the term, "newborn" in neonatology. Biologically, this entails a period of 0-4 weeks: the ductus Botalli closes, lung tissues open, the foramen ovale (opening in the septum secundum of the heart) closes. Often, the term, "newborn" is extended to refer to a period of up to three months. This period, however, does not have a biological basis and can be stretched to six months or a year, the definition being used to find more time for the eventual ending of a life.

Since the seventies, possibilities for prenatal diagnosis have multiplied. Those were the years in which personal autonomy and self-determination took root in society. There is an illusion that humans are becoming increasingly independent. You don't need to go to the office to work, you can work from your house; shopping is not necessary, the computer delivers the items to the front door. Having a car frees you from using a train or bus, with a credit card you can pay anywhere in the world, the cellular phone makes you free as a bird. Prenatal testing can free you from embryonic risks and insurance softens the cruel blows of fate. Along the same line, people create new living arrangements, follow their own choices and don't allow themselves to be "dictated" regarding their actions, feelings, and morals. All of this gives the illusion of not-needing-anybody, of independence, of autonomy to the bitter end. This is an illusion, since in reality that autonomy is only possible thanks to a fine web of many invisible strings to which more and more people are connected. If this web falters, you are left empty-handed and are given over body and bones to your fellowman from whom you thought you had been freed. To prevent such a state of dependence, humans are assumed to have the right to end their own lives. In the Netherlands, this right was advocated first by professor H. Drion. Since then, the "Drion pill" (available on prescription in order to decide the moment of your death yourself) has become a widely advocated concept. Dutch actress Emmy Lopes at age 77 founded an organization which claims that everyone should have the right to take one's life and to have access to all necessary measures to do so.

In our present-day health care system, "health problems" are often determined by our "health expectations". This has led to an ongoing expansion of the number of indications for genetic counselling and prenatal diagnostics, in turn leading to an increased amount of prenatal selectivity. The combination of medical-technical and societal developments contributed to the acceptance by the medical sciences of the choice of ending the life of the unborn if handicapped. The wish to dispose of the human embryo is the same as giving in to the desire to choose whom we want to be our equals. It would mean that we ourselves want to manage the limits of a whole of which we are a part. It would mean the denial of the existence of our fellowman, more than that: we would deny that the existence of the other ultimately is the basis for the possibility of our own existence (ontological solidarity). If we do not honour human life from the first moment it comes into being, then we are refusing to recognize that we ourselves are humans only because of other human beings whom we never chose.

Already prior to birth, the verdict has been made that the death of a (wanted) child with mental retardation is better than its staying alive.[19] This verdict has influenced how we view people with handicaps *after* their birth. This moral verdict illustrates the close link between our normative view of man (or "normative anthropology") and our moral convictions and decisions (cf. the elaboration on ethics and worldview in the Introduction). A view of man comprises the image which people have both of themselves and of others; it forms the point of reference from which people understand and listen to each other.

5. APPLIED CRITERIA AND ETHICS

Facts and values, medical-technical findings, and normative decisions are strongly tied together in our day to day health care. In order to stay on top of the complexities, objective criteria and score-charts are used. No matter how objective they seem to be, these score-charts and criteria do not provide substantive clues as to what should be done. We cannot solve moral problems by using check-lists only. We need substantive moral criteria.

In order to provide a more substantive criterion, many people make use of the terms, "livable" and "unlivable". However, this has some disadvantages. As a descriptive term, an "unlivable life" is comparable to a rectangular circle: after all, the patient *is* alive! Moreover, these terms often have a discriminative tone. Use of the term "unlivable" often functions as a kind of final verdict which subsequently takes away all hope from a class of patients and their parents by implicitly denying them the right to further assistance. Health care is assumed to be "good" only as long as it adds life to the days of a person, rather than adding days to a person's life. The term "unlivable" has the implicit normative suggestion that the life of the person concerned should be ended. In practice, therefore, the use of this term contributes to the problem rather than solving it.

Whether or not the life of a patient is meaningful and worth living, does not only depend on the good and bad that lies ahead of him. It also depends on the meaning and value that those involved give to his or her life. How we attribute meaning to the lives of others is influenced by our own perspective on life, by what we expect for ourselves, by what we hope for and fear. The concept of "good and bad" has a moral and also a spiritual dimension; it falls outside of the realm of the medical profession. The future of the child with serious (mental) retardation and the future of societal solidarity are not two separate issues: this future is dependent on whether or not there are enough people who view life with a child with a handicap as a life worth living.[20]

On April 9, 1997, the European Parliament adopted a resolution that honors the rights of the individual in the European Union. The resolution mentions some points that concern people with mental retardation. Under the heading, "the right to live and die with dignity", we read

> . . . urges that euthanasia at the cost of the handicapped, chronic coma-patients, handicapped infants, and elderly be prohibited; urges member-states to create circumstances that allow the dying to be attended to in a dignified fashion in the end phase of life (point 18).

The preceding point 17 is as follows:

> . . . confirms that the right to life also includes the right to health-care and therefore also the right to treatment, and that this right must apply to all persons, regardless of their status, health, gender, ethnic background, colour of their skin, age, or religion.

The next point 19:

> confirms that all living persons in the [European] Union have the need to live without fear for their personal safety.

Two other interesting points are point 9 (concerning a new article 6.a in the Treaty of the European Union regarding prohibition of discrimination on grounds of a number of characteristics, including having a handicap), and point 122 (firming up the basic law of equal opportunity and non-discrimination for people with a handicap in the policy of the European Community). The agreement of the European Union does not provide the European Community with any authority in the medical-ethical sector. The European Parliament can merely give an opinion regarding medical-ethical issues, possibly influencing certain policies by voicing concerns.

In 1996, the Finnish Liberal Seppe Pelttari drew up a report about bio-ethics, which led to a resolution that protects the rights of the individual and preserves human dignity in biological and medical practices (accepted on Friday morning, September 20, 1996, when the quorum of 100 members of Parliament was no longer present). In article 6 of this resolution are listed regulations for medical trials with people who are deemed incompetent, regulations that preserve indisputable human dignity, and regulations that prohibit discriminatory measures with regard to people with handicaps. Medical research involving a subject deemed incompetent must only be allowed in exceptional circumstances: (1) his legal guardian gives free and informed consent keeping in account all legal rights, (2) the considered action is strongly related to this person's medical issues, (3) the study cannot be performed by using competent subjects, and (4) the nature of the research might have a positive effect on the health of the subject. Human worth is indivisible; there must not be any discriminating regulations for people with a handicap; only the making of decisions in name of the incompetent can be regulated by law, and the same criteria ought to count as in the decisions of the competent.

The terms, "prevention" and "selection" are at times carelessly interchanged. The prevention of handicaps (when possible) belongs to the realm of medical practice. Since nearly all mothers are vaccinated against Rubella, children are no longer born blind because of a congenital German Measles infection. This vaccination falls in the category of primary prevention: the condition or handicap is prevented. A therapeutic abortion performed because prenatal exams revealed the presence of a Rubella infection, is usually referred to under the veil of "secondary prevention", when in actuality it is negative selection: the natural birth of a person who carries a (potential) handicap has been hindered. Having a handicap can be meaningful in a human life. Where possible, handicaps are prevented or solutions are looked for (not wanting to prevent, or even look for a handicap is pathological). The choice against handicaps, however, must not lead to a choice against the *person* with a handicap. Of course, sometimes a premature birth is induced in order to save the life of the infant and spare it from possible handicaps.

In the brochure, *Equal Opportunities*, the Dutch Federation of Parent Associations (FVO) gives her vision on medical practices with newborns who have mental handicaps.[21] In the brochure, the Federation reacts to the report *To Act or Not to Act* of the Dutch Association for Paediatrics. The parents object to the false objectivity and the vagueness of the criteria, and also to the negative picture that is drawn of the person with a handicap. A child with mental retardation has the same right to life, and thus to the same life-saving medical measures around the birth and thereafter, as any other child. The diagnosis of "mental retardation" is not a criterion in and of itself in determining the type and amount of care the child receives; medical practice is built on the assumption that each individual has the right to life. Treating pain and other symptoms is essential to meaningful medical care, even without a therapeutic perspective. Sometimes it speeds up the dying process, but this accepted side-effect is not the goal.

Expectations as to the future development of the child cannot and must not play a role in choosing to start or terminate an intervention, according to these parents. Because society often has little notion of the great shift in nature and measure of existing handicaps, it misses sufficient insight in the possibilities of people with mental retardation. People with mental retardation get ill just like any other person, but they are not "patients" by definition. It seems to me that the Federation of Parent Associations is too absolute regarding development opportunities, because expectations concerning developmental prospects should, in my opinion, play a role in the decision whether treatment is meaningful or not (*cf.* chapter eight). Moreover, the quality and availability of care facilities should never be allowed to be the predictor of future "quality of life" — a term which, according to the parents, shouldn't belong in medical vocabulary. Abstaining[22], the decision of the attending physician to cease treatment, can only be based on medical criteria (i.e., medical benefit and proportionality) and should never be based on a judgment whether the life of a person is meaningful.[23]

When in doubt, what do we do? Thanks to medical technology, much suffering can be prevented and more people can experience joyful lives. However, technology brings ambivalence and is full of risk: it leads to a sense of alienation and poses a threat to the human nature of health care. As medical technology has reached a place of dominance in the health care sector, the basis for medical ethics has changed accordingly. The dominating picture in current health care ethics is that of the self-determining individual. Since people with serious mental retardation lack the ability to self-determination, this view implies an attack on the worth of the person and a loss of moral value in life. When the care recipient does not have an own (autonomous) life-perspective, a value crisis develops in the provision of care: the more that "natural" limitations create a loss of autonomy in a person, the scarcer becomes the value of his or her care. A care ethic based on such a reductionistic viewpoint leaves no moral stronghold in situations where limitations of autonomy cannot be removed. If one yet wants to put an emphasis on "people with possibilities" (terminology used by the Dutch Federation of Parent' Associations) when dealing with people with mental retardation, the emphasis of health care ethics on autonomy and self-determination is brought out even more: the "possibilities" that come in the picture are reduced to how much of a will a person with mental retardation has. On what grounds are moral considerations in health care based, when it is not or not completely clear what exactly the person's will is?

Three classic proverbs that each physician has grown up with are: never kill, *primum non nocere*, and *in dubio abstine*. In other words: a life should not be ended, prevention of damage should take first place, and if in doubt of the results of a treatment, the physician should abstain. In present time we seem to say, *in dubio fac* (always resuscitate and use technical supports to the utmost) and afterwards, let die if needed. The Dutch ethicist H.M. Dupuis operates two "completely reasonable and arguable strategies" to prevent damaging medical intervention in the case of incompetence (coma): a) do not treat, unless there is an expression of will and unless it is based on a clear indication; b) institute experimental treatment and, if the treatment turns out to be damaging, actively pursue death. "Because of a certain interpretation of the law, this is impossible in the United States as well as in the Netherlands, to our detriment." However, this practice is now no longer out of the question in the Netherlands. Professor Dupuis has discovered three problems in the second option, of which one is of a psychological nature: when one first has fought for a life, it is difficult to switch over to pursuing death. When the results of an intensive intervention are disappointing, it is argued, physicians must have a way to undo these negative results. As long as careful considerations are made, every outcome is acceptable. As a result, medical developments are uncontrolled and any treatment can be initiated. After all, isn't there always a way out if the intervention doesn't lend its desired results?

6. CONCLUSION

In this contribution, my intention was to give a brief introduction to the field of neonatology, a field which is complex and sometimes gray, which contains numerous pitfalls, and where choices concerning life and death frequently occur. In times when the child was considered a gift of God, the question of quality did not play a role: a child with a handicap was a test of God, who was not asked any questions, for His ways were impenetrable. It has become a different issue, however, now that science can help us "produce" a child. It belongs to the logic of making that the product has to meet the demands for quality. A sound product receives the label of quality. Is it not inconceivable, after all, that medicine would deliver sick and handicapped children?

In their professions, Christian health care providers recognize the experience of Ambroise Paré (1510-1590), a famous sixteenth century surgeon and obstetrician: "*je le pans et Dieu le gurit*" — I bandaged his wounds, and God healed him. As physician and army surgeon of king François I of Valois (ruled from 1515-1547), he marches into the city of Turin with the conquering French army.[24] A flood of sympathy overwhelms Paré when he hears the bones of corpses and the dying crunch under the hooves of the horses. When he observes an old soldier cutting the throats of three of his already dying colleagues, the problem of ending someone's life becomes literally clear-cut.[25]

Christian care provision is inspired by the parable of the good Samaritan.[26] If medicine is truly *medicina ministra misericordiae*, servant of mercy, then we can say in the words of Paré: "*guérir quelquefois, soulager souvent, consoler toujours*": heal sometimes, alleviate often, console always.

NOTES

1 From the ciconiidae family; the Dutch name for stork, "ooievaar", comes from the thirteenth century word "odevare" or "bringer of luck": a heron type of bird (white feathers with jet black flight feathers and long, bright red beak/legs, flies slowly and calmly (with a stretched out and slightly bent down neck), walks with careful steps and nests on roofs, chimneys, haystacks and at times in trees.

2 Apart from that, there is a growing acceptance of life-terminating interventions on incompetent patients. In the Netherlands, an estimated 1.000 times a year, life-termination takes place without explicit request. G.H. Blijham and J.J.M. van Delden, "Actieve levensbeëindiging bij wilsonbekwame volwassenen: Aandachtspunten voor zorgvuldig handelen" (Active Life Termination of Incompetent Adults: Criteria for Careful Decisions), in: *Medisch Contact* Vol 54, nr. 10 (1999), pp. 344-347. Active life-termination without request seems to be contrary to article 2 of the European Declaration of Human Rights and fundamental Freedom. A Dutch District Court recently decided that these cases belong in the category, "emergencies" and can therefore not be overruled by European rules.

3 J. Janssens, "Verloskunde en gynaecologie in de laatste 40 jaar" (Obstetrics and Gynaecology in the Past Forty Years), *Nederlands Tijdschrift voor Geneeskunde*, Vol. 141, no. 1 (1997), pp. 26-32.

4 T.W.J. Schulpen and A. van Enk, "Mortaliteit naar etniciteit bij kinderen in Nederland" (Mortality and Ethnicity of Children in the Netherlands), *Nederlands Tijdschrift voor Geneeskunde*, Vol. 140 (1996), pp. 2489-92.

5 H.H. de Haan, "De pathofysiologie van perinatale asfyxie en cerebrale beschadiging" (The Pathophysiology of Perinatal Asphyxia and Cerebral Trauma), *Nederlands Tijdschrift voor Geneeskunde*, Vol. 139, no. 33 (1995), pp. 1673-6.

6 Premature infants (gestation of 26-32 weeks) and immature infants (gestation of 24-26 weeks). *Cf.* M.C. Allen, P.K. Donohue, and A.E. Dusman, "The limit of viability — neonatal outcome of infants born at 22 to 25 weeks' gestation", *New England Journal of Medicine*, Nr. 329 (1993), pp. 1597-1601.

7 The division of neonatology is subdivided into intensive care (in cases of serious threat or needed support in one or more vital functions, including respiratory, cardiac, circulatory, and excretory systems), high care (nursing of seriously ill neonates without direct threat to vital functions) and medium care (newborns who do not need 24 hour per day observation).

8 The Royal Dutch Association of Medicine wrote the discussion report, *Levensbeëindigend handelen bij wilsonbekwame patiënten. Deel I: zwaar-defecte pasgeborenen* (*Life-terminating Interventions with Incompetent Patients, Part 1: Severely Defective Newborns*). Utrecht: Koninklijke Nederlandsche Maatschappij tot Bevordering der Geneeskunst, 1990. The Dutch Association for Paediatrics issued *Doen of laten? Grenzen van het medisch handelen in neonatologie* (*To Act or Not to Act: Limits of Medical Care in Neonatology*). Utrecht: Nederlandse Vereniging voor Kindergeneeskunde, 1992.

9 M.J.K. de Kleine, R. de Leeuw, L.A.A. Kollée, and H.M. Berger, "Voortzetten of staken van levensverlengend handelen bij pasgeborenen: een onderzoek in 4 centra voor neonatale intensieve zorg" (Continuing or Withdrawal of Life Sustaining Treatment of Newborns: a Survey in Four Centers of Intensive Neonatal Care), *Nederlands Tijdschrift voor Geneeskunde,* Vol. 137, no.10 (1993), pp. 496-9.

10 *Cf.* T.L. Beauchamp and J.F. Childress, *Principles of Biomedical Ethics*. New York, Oxford: Oxford University Press, 1983, pp. 14-7; 131-2.

11 W.W. Eigner, H. Knol, Th. Neuer-Miebach, M.H. Rioux, C. van de Vate, and M. Bunch, *Just Technology? From Principles to Practice in Bio-ethical Issues.* Brussels: International League of Societies for Persons with Mental Handicaps/ L'Institut Roeher Institute, 1994.

12 H.M. Evenhuis, R.A. van Beek, K. Cuperus-Suithof, C.H.A. van Schie, and F. Schuckinck Kool, "Medische zorg voor verstandelijk gehandicapten: een eigen vakgebied" (Medical Care for People with Mental Retardation as a Profession of Its Own), in: *Medisch Contact*, Vol. 49, no. 42 (1994), pp. 1317-8.

13 C. van de Vate, "Parental Ethics," in J.M. Berg *et al.*, *Report on the European workshop "Bio-ethics and Mental Handicap."* Utrecht: Bishop Bekkers Foundation, 1992.

14 Under commission of the association 's Heeren Loo, the Center for Bio-ethics and Health Law of the University Utrecht researched medical decisions regarding the ending of life in healthcare of people with mental retardation. G.M.W. van Thiel, A.K. Huibers, and K. de Haan, *Met zorg besluiten: beslissingen rond het levenseinde in de zorg voor mensen met een verstandelijke handicap* (Deciding Wisely: End of Life Decisions in the Care or People with Mental Retardation). Assen: Van Gorcum, 1997. In this study, 89 physicians reported a total of 859 cases of death. In several situations, physicians did not discuss their medical decisions surrounding the death with the parents, sometimes not even with anyone. There were four cases in which life was ended without request (0.5%). The study indicated that the active ending of life within the health care sector occurs one to two times per year. (Cf. J. Stolk, "Euthanasie bei geistig Behinderten: eine Bewertung der aktuellen Euthanasie-Diskussion in den Niederlanden" (Euthanasia and People with Mental Retardation: An Evaluation of the Recent Discussion in the Netherlands), *Geistige Behinderung*, Vol. 29, no. 4 (1990), pp. 386-93.

15 A.Th.G. van Gennep, "Wat is goed doen? 'Levensperspectief' voor een pasgeborene met een ernstige handicap" (What is Beneficence? 'Life-Perspective' of Newborns with Serious Handicaps), in: T. van Willigenburg and W. Kuis, *Op de grens van leven en dood: afzien van behandelen en levensbeëindiging in de neonatologie* (On the Verge of Life and Death: Refraining from Treatment and Life Termination in Neonatology). Assen: Van Gorcum, 1995, pp. 42-51.

16 H.A.M. Alpine, "Geen uitzicht op menswaardig bestaan" (No Prospects for a Liveable Life), *Tijdschrift voor Geneeskunde en Ethiek*, Vol. 5, No. 1 (1995), pp. 23-9.

17 *Cf.* baby K. and Willy in chapter 8.

18 *Cf.* J.J. Rotteveel, R.A. Mullaart, F.J.M. Gabreëls, and J.J. van Overbeeke, "Actieve levensbeëindiging bij pasgeborenen met spina bifida?" (Life Termination of Newborns with Bifid Spine?), *Nederlands Tijdschrift voor Geneeskunde*, Vol. 140, No. 6 (1996), pp. 323-4.

19 *Cf.* Chapter 9.

20 J.S. Reinders, *Moeten wij gehandicapt leven voorkomen? Ethische implicaties van beslissingen over kinderen met een aangeboren of erfelijke handicap* (Should We Prevent Handicapped Life? Moral Implications of Decisions about Children with Congenital or Hereditary Conditions). Utrecht: Nederlandse Vereniging voor Bio-ethiek, 1996. According to Reinders, judgments about the future of a child with a handicap are rooted in our personal identity. On the basis of how we understand our own humanity, would we not come to the conclusion that the existence of people with mental retardation should have a quality that signifies a good life?

21 *Gelijke kansen: medisch handelen rond pasgeborenen met een (verstandelijke) handicap.* Utrecht: Vereniging Federatie van Ouderverenigingen, 1993.

22 Derived from the Latin word, "abstinentia" = abstinence; not using (anymore), not giving something to someone (anymore). This idea cannot be associated with actively terminating someone's life. Further treatment is abandoned because at the patient's request or because the treatment offers no chance medically. Meanwhile, nursing and general care are provided as usual.

23 U. Eibach, *Medizin und Menschenwürde. Ethische Probleme in der Medizin aus christlicher Sicht.* (Medicine and Human Dignity: Moral Problems in Medicine from a Christian Perspective). Wuppertal: Brockhaus, 1997[5]

24 G.A. Lindeboom, *Euthanasie in historisch perspectief* (Euthanasia: a Historical Overview). Amsterdam: Rodopi, 1978.

25 Two people, deeply moved by human suffering, react in two completely different ways. In a way, these two figures in the dimmed stable of Turin have a symbolic significance. The soldier appears out of society and immediately acts, deeply moved, with deliberateness of mind. But behind the appearance of the no less sympathetic Paré, Professor Lindeboom sees as it were the face of Hippocrates (460-375 BC). It is in his name that one finds the 25 century old creed of physicians, which states without hesitation the primary clause: "I will not administer a deadly remedy to anyone, even not upon his request, and will not offer any advice in that nature." These words want to give solidity to the conscience of the physician that at times can face doubts in the face of unexpected situations.

26 The Bible, Luke 10:25-37.

ULRICH EIBACH

CHAPTER 7

MEDICAL TECHNIQUE AND OUR COPING WITH SUFFERING:

Prenatal Diagnosis as an Example

1. INTRODUCTION

Medical ethics and, more generally, the objectives of medicine are in a crisis. This crisis is caused by two factors: recent progresses in medical techniques, and the increasing plurality in ways of life and in moral values in western industrialized countries since the nineteen-sixties.

2. CHANGES IN SOCIAL VALUES AND MEDICAL ETHICS

As a consequence of the rapid changes in societal circumstances, we see a liberation of the human individual from his social constraints and an increase in individual self-realization.[1] At the core of this change is a quest for autonomy and for the satisfaction of individual needs, especially needs for a happy life, for which health and the absence of suffering are supposed to be the most basic prerequisites. In the traditional Hippocratic oath, there is no mention of the autonomy of the individual patient. In contrast, the will of the patient has today become the foremost action guiding standard for physicians.

This over-valuation of the autonomous human self is based on the assumption that human life has to be the object of human control, to the effect that it is fully defined and directed by human conceptions. This has several consequences. First, there is a decreasing preparedness and capacity to accept and come to terms with unwanted severe suffering or disabilities as a "destiny" or as "God's will". Similarly, there is a decreasing societal tolerance to accept human beings that do not fill the prevailing conceptions of a "normal" or "happy" life, beings whose existence form a continuous and often severe burden for society as a whole.

Many people would argue that our conceptions about prenatal diagnosis and selection, as well as our conceptions about euthanasia, do not have any link with the assumptions which formed the basis for the criminal acts of German physicians during the Nazi-period. A comparison of German ideology and praxis before and

Joop Stolk, Theo A. Boer & Ruth Seldenrijk (eds.). Meaningful Care, 101—112

during World War Two, and recent tendencies in the health care sector in western countries, however, shows some parallels.[2] National Socialism put into practice what social-darwinistic and other scholars at the beginning of the twentieth century propagated as a rational and even natural scientific (i.e., evolutionistic) ethics.[3] This heritage which is widespread in the western industrialized world, was summarized by the criminal law expert Karl Binding and psychiatrist Alfred Hoche in 1920 in their concerted book "The Admission of the Destruction of Unworthy Life".[4] The theoretical nucleus of this writing consisted primarily of the allegation that an individual human being looses the right to legal protection to the degree to which he becomes a continuous and heavy burden for his society, and cannot enjoy his own life any more; it consists, secondly, in the assumption — with which later in time Nazi-doctors tried to justify their criminal acts in court procedures — that there are too few medical, personal, and financial resources. In light of this, they argue, we need to concentrate our efforts on those who have a reasonable chance of rehabilitation, so that they will not be a continuous burden for the state. Those, however, for whom this goal cannot be accomplished, should be freed from their existence; instead of giving them meaningless care, we should care for those who can enjoy their own lives and who have a certain utility for society. This ideology, therefore, only allowed these alternatives: "healing", or "killing".[5]

The well-known physician Viktor von Weizsäcker published a critique of Nazi-medicine.[6] In this study, von Weizsäcker has successfully shown that the fierceful battle of medicine against diseases and death, and the destruction of the "incurable", can be seen as two sides of the same coin, i.e., the glorification of health and of an earthly life which is free from suffering.

Disabled, incurably ill, and persons in need of continuous care, disturb the mistaken assumption that humans can gain full control over their lives, that a "whole" world can be accomplished, and that life can be lived in full and unrubbed autonomy. When it becomes clear that we cannot free the ill and the disabled of their suffering, only one way seems to be let open: to terminate their lives, in order to remove the suffering alongside with their very lives.

The ethos of a radical autonomy, of absolute self-determination, and the delusion that life can be put in the service of human plans, originate from the same ideological source, according to which humans are the self-appointed almighty rulers of life. Both deny the status of createdness, of continuous dependence on factors beyond human control, nature, and God, and they deny that all creation is submitted to the powers of disease and death.[7] They therefore lack an ethics in which terms such as "giving up" and "endurance" have a place. Instead, this ethics is an ethos of active cultivation, of accomplishing, according to which the individual human person is master of nature. It is an "ethics of power", which attempts to hide its powerlessness in the face of diseases and death by the use of power. There can be no "let go", no inner reconciliation with God's will or with human destiny. It principally denies the fact that, in our world, not human freedom and power, but disease and death win the victory. By this victory, the power of the human individual is dethroned, albeit without making human life unworthy and unlivable.

3. CONSEQUENCES OF THE CHANGES IN VALUES FOR MEDICAL PRACTICE

As a consequence of the increasing plurality in worldviews and of the progress of medical knowledge and skills, the medical ethos which traditionally focused on care has become more and more problematic. The solution has been sought in exalting "Patient Autonomy" as the highest moral principle. Alongside the individualization of worldviews, the introduction of almost every new medical technique is legitimated with reference to the wishes of the medical consumers. How, it is argued, can we deny some the legitimate claim to get what they desire? Should they not be able to have access to new techniques, as long as those who have moral objections are free to refuse? Those who do not wish to make use of new procedures themselves, are wrong in willing to prevent others make use of them. The fact is, of course, that support can be found or aggregated for almost any medical procedure, even for cloning human beings, and that basically any medical intervention can be justified by referring to the wishes of individuals. If this line is accepted, there is no point in critically evaluating the objectives of medical progress at all, because these objectives are fully identical to the individual needs of health care receivers which, in turn, are defined by the wish for a life as healthy and as happy as possible. So we are left with a medicine which offers any services as long as they can be accomplished and as long as someone is sufficiently interested in them. Such a medicine will ultimately not have any ethical boundaries, neither in the conduction nor in the application of research, for human needs for health, prosperity and happiness are just as infinite as the scientific quest to gain control over life.

A medical ethics, which does not have a substantial *ethos* of caring for the weak as its basis, but which instead conceives the justification of its scientific and therapeutic practice solely or primarily by referring to the autonomy and claims of individual human beings, will ultimately not have any lasting boundaries to the urges of the medical researchers and the expectations of the consumers alike. We therefore need an ethos of care. An ethos of care can best be understood as an ethics of existence, i.e., concerned with life in its most comprehensive sense. An ethos of care formulates values which are crucial for our experiences of meaning. It comprises daily-life experiences of care and acceptance. No doubt, respect for autonomy is one of the elements which lead to experiences of meaning. However, when the possibility to express one's will is not, or not yet present, on whose autonomy should medical decisions be based? Characteristic of an ethos of care is acceptance of the fact that we share our existence with others. We are all dependent upon our acceptance by others, and *vice versa*.

An ethos of care must not be understood as a license to go on treating and "caring" for as long as you please. Not only is the care-giver bound to stay within the limits of what is medically meaningful; an ethos of care also implies respect for the needs, the interests, the well-being and the biography of the care-receiver. Moreover, the care-giver needs to have insight in his own moral presuppositions; not knowing oneself carries the risk of imposing one's own norms on others.[8]

An ethics of autonomy which is not grounded in an ethos of care and of the protection of human life, will only offer protection as long as people have the opportunity and the strength to defend their own interests. This kind of an ethics of autonomy, which is not rooted in and submitted to an ethos of care, will end up as an ethics of the fittest. Such an ethics without care is forceful only as long as it promotes a reverence for one's own life and for one's own happiness. At the same time, it will provide a threat to the life protection and right to life of the weakest.[9]

4. THE MEDICAL PREVENTION OF THE BIRTH OF DISEASED AND DISABLED LIFE

New medical procedures to prevent the birth of diseased and disabled persons will only be used in societies, in which the termination of a pregnancy is not a legal offence. It is my contention that, in the case of abortion, the main conflict concerns the desire of the parents for individual self-fulfillment, and the protection of unborn life. Concerns for the well-being of the future child as a reason for abortion — "being unwanted will make the child unhappy" — seem to be secondary to the self-fulfillment of the parents. According to German law, abortion is legal when living with a child presents an unbearable burden for the future mother. The basic moral notion here is the tolerability, according to which the life protection of the child-in-the-making is submitted to the need of the adults for a happy life. When even the prospect of a healthy baby presents an unbearable loss of life quality, how much more will the prospect of living with a child who is handicapped be conceived as an unbearable burden.

Most people who volunteer to see a genetic counsellor, do not wish to have a child with a handicap, so that the wish to prevent the birth of such a child is virtually always the basic motivation behind such a session. Not without reason, the counsellors try to retrieve themselves to a "value-neutral", medically informing counselling, and avoid to refrain from giving a moral judgment, as they would like to leave such a judgment to the parents only.[10] One of the advantages of this practice may be that the suspicion is avoided that the counsellor is pursuing preventive-eugenic objectives with his counselling. Moreover, such a non-directive attitude fits the societal trend to promote the making of autonomous decisions. By a lack of societal and medical consensus, the individual is expected to "autonomously" give the last word. Is it really so coincidental that the individual will most probably decide along his own inclinations, as well as in line with the prevailing social expectations?

One of the risks of the practice of genetic counselling is that it tends to focus only on the situation of the individual. This puts a serious constraint upon the ethical perspective, as it is mainly concerned about the question whether life with a child who is handicapped is a tolerable burden for the parents. In a moral evaluation, however, there is more at stake than only the destiny of one or more individuals. One also has to deal with the consequences of such a choice for society as a whole and for the whole system of values and norms, as new medical procedures do have a much larger impact than is often acknowledged. The use of genetic and prenatal testing procedures, for example, may have a bearing on the lives of existing people with a handicap, and on the attitude of others to them.

4.1. Genome Analysis and Prenatal Diagnosis between the Protection and Selection of Life

In no other area of medicine is there such a tremendous gap between diagnostic skills and possibilities for therapy as in the area of prenatal diagnostics. A deliberate choice is being made in favor of a diagnosis without any serious chance for therapy for the diagnosed "object". In medicine, this is a *novum*, as diagnostic devices and procedures are normally only justified when they provide a basis to serve the well-being of the diagnosed "object". In the practice of prenatal diagnosis, the finding of a disease or handicap will almost necessarily lead to abortion. Instead of receiving therapy, the bearer of the disease will most probably be killed.[11]

The prenatal diagnosis of a non-curable disease or handicap ultimately provokes human beings to make judgments about the value of life, judgments so severe that the life of the child depends on it. This presents a second basic novelty of these methods. In effect, the most poignant reason for applying and using these diagnostic procedures is the intention to prevent the birth of diseased children. This can almost only be accomplished by killing the fetus. It is my conviction that prenatal diagnosis would almost certainly be superfluous when parents would be prepared to accept a child with a handicap. As this preparedness is widely absent in our western societies, there is a great need for what I would call "Lethal Diagnostics". We see here that the development and availability of such techniques provokes new needs and it will continue to do so, as the range of diagnosable diseases gets larger and larger. Until these procedures were developed, the ethical challenge was to come to terms with the occurrence of an unavoidable destiny — or, at least, to tolerate it. Instead, we now have options to use which for the unborn human being with a disease almost certainly imply death. This illustrates quite convincingly our propensity to accept any technique which promises to keep us clear from the risks of unwanted suffering.

To be sure, not everyone will agree with the contention that prenatal diagnosis doesn't allow therapeutic possibilities, that such diagnosis provides the basis for judgments about the value of life of the unborn child, and that we actually exert a form of "prenatal euthanasia". Some would argue, for example, that we should widen our definition of the "therapeutic object" as to even comprise the social context of the child, such as the parents, other relatives, or even society as a whole. In this option, the terms "health", "happiness", and "tolerability" refer to a wider circle than the child or, for that matter its parents. The question, it is said, is: how does the birth of such a child affect the happiness of a larger community? Such an extension of the term, "therapeutic object", however, presents a novelty in medical ethics, as it has almost exclusively been used to refer to an individual subject, not to a social body.

Nevertheless, there should, of course, also be a concern for the well-being of those who surround the future child. There is a point in conceiving parents and others as therapeutic objects, because the person with a handicap will be especially and continuously dependent upon social networks and upon the care of his relatives. Marriages and families may well suffer from such a burden. It is in order to prevent such a predicament, that abortions are being performed. It can, however, be seriously doubted whether the burdens of having a child with a handicap are a sufficient moral justification for ending its life during the beginning of the pregnancy. If this is the case, we might also ask why such a predicament would not also warrant the killing of a child in a later phase. When we extend the concept of "therapeutic object" to the family, the danger is a slippery slope: why not conceive "society" as a therapeutic object, which should be protected from having to carry the burdens of caring for people who are handicapped? In western countries, there is already a widespread opinion that it is irresponsible for future parents to refuse the use of genetic testing and prenatal diagnostic procedures, as this places too much of a burden upon society as a whole. In the end, this implies that, again, the value of life and the right to life are made subject to the burdens and benefits that it presents for society. Human life looses the privilege of legal protection as soon as its burdens exceed its benefits for society.[12] It is on this point that we should be especially cautious not to repeat the mistakes of the past.

Such and similar justifications for "selecting out" people with a handicap may gain social and political credit as the economic pressure in health care and the social sector increases, in combination with growing uncertainty about what establishes the value and dignity of people who are severely handicapped or incurably ill. The fear seems warranted that prenatal diagnosis will lead to discrimination and selection of entire categories of human beings. Alongside the development of genetic and other testing methods, it seems unavoidable that the inhuman fiction of a world without serious diseases and disorders will gain support, so that the social tolerance of persons who are seriously handicapped and incurable will show a steady decrease. Thus, the "urge for a healthy society" poses a threat to the right to life, and develops into a tendency to sort out the weakest.[13]

4.2. Predictive Medicine — Prevention by Selection?

Genetic screening not only implies the diagnosis of diseases and handicaps already present before, during, or soon after the birth of a child, but also of disorders which will develop in the course of its later life.

Through the possibilities of "predictive medicine", our whole concept of disease tends to change. Diseased is not only the person whose physical, psychological, or mental well-being is actually affected by a disorder, but also the one whose genetic structure displays the *disposition* to develop certain diseases. Whether this person will actually develop the disease, or will actually live his entire life without any visible manifestation of it, seems to be of minor importance. The extension of our conception of diseases from a physical-organic to a genetic level renders healthy persons into diseased persons. Even the lives of the potentially ill will, however well they may function on a physical level, be seen to be of less value and therefore not have the full right to protection. The urge for health and for the prevention of diseases for the well-being of society as a whole, will lead to an unpredictable and hideous extension of the group of those whose lives are considered unwanted on the basis of insufficient genetic quality.

It is not the intention to say that an ethos of care justifies any medical treatment of unborns and newborns as long as it stems from a "caring attitude". Some infants are in such a condition that medical treatment to "save this life" is meaningless. Children with Patau's syndrome, for example, have a life-expectancy of days rather than weeks; 70% of the infants die within the first month after birth. Patau's syndrome is characterized by multiple serious deformities. In this and similar cases — depending on the seriousness of the child's condition —, treatment will normally be confined to palliative care, without intentionally causing death or speeding the process of dying.

4.3. From Prenatal Diagnosis to "Euthanasia"

That there is a blurred transition from prenatal diagnosis to "early euthanasia", is demonstrated when the performing of abortion leads to the birth of a living baby. In Germany, this situation occurs increasingly since the law on abortion was altered in 1996. Since then, the special embryopathic indication for termination of a pregnancy has disappeared as an independent category and resides from then on as one of the "medical indications". This change, which came about on the urgent request of organisations of people with a handicap and of the churches, reflects Article 2 of the German Constitution which forbids the discrimination of people with a handicap.[14] The change intended to put a halt to a discriminating practice in which handicapped fetuses could be aborted without further motivation, and would grant both diseased and healthy children the same right to life. In practice, this has come to mean that no longer a defect of the child, but only an "unbearable burden" for the woman (parents) counts as a valid reason for an abortion. Since this "indication" resides under the medical indications, one can easily overlook the fact that the physical life of the mother is usually not threatened at all. Even more important is that since the German law was changed, there is no longer a limited period within which abortion is allowed. Instead of the former limitation of 22-24 weeks for an abortion on embryopathic indication, the present medical indication does not put any temporal limitation at all.

As a consequence, an increasing number of aborted children that come into the world are alive and viable, but are denied the necessary care to stay alive. Since the actual intention behind the abortion is that the child will be stillborn (or, more precisely, will get killed), many consider the viability of the child as an undesirable side-effect — or "complication" — of the abortion. This "complication" imposes a serious mental and moral burden, not only on the woman who requested the abortion, but also for all the persons who are professionally involved in this happening: physicians, midwives, nurses. The "complication" of a fetus which proves to be viable presents a hitherto unsolved legal problem. Such children are, according to the law in most Western countries (including Germany), "persons", towards whom others have a caring duty. In order to circumvent these problems, some hospitals have decided to kill the child before it is taken out of the womb. Others have serious difficulties with this form of "active" killing. In some cases, a fetus with considerable chances of survival is denied medically meaningful care.[15] That this situation is morally problematic, is demonstrated by the fact that newborns of the same age with similar health problems and with an often even smaller chance for survival, receive all the necessary care and treatment in the Intensive Care Unit. Crucial in the decision whether to treat or to kill by denying proper care is ultimately an act of will, namely, whether a child may live or not. In the first case, the "medical complication" consists in the disorder and the premature birth, whereas in the latter case it consists in the being alive of the baby. This clearly indicates the difficulty of identifying a clear distinction between a prenatal killing (abortion), postnatal killing ("early euthanasia"), infanticide, and the killing of adults.

If we make moral decisions on the basis of whether something might be "unbearable", it is — as Singer and others before him have made clear — inconsistent to confine the right to get killed to a rather dubitable criterion of viability outside the uterus, in combination with a reasonably early diagnosis of a defect. If something is "unbearable", it will be so even after this particular stage in the life development has passed. Now that life in its early stages has become subject to human disposition, and now that society has got used to certain forms of prenatal euthanasia and early euthanasia by referring to a possible "unbearable burden", the moment will come sooner or later that even other life phases, particularly the end of life, will be made subject to autonomous or paternalistic decisions to end someone's life. The only reasonable ground for the decision whether someone should live or die, will ultimately be the human will — whether one's own will, or, as a consequence of increasing social and economic pressure, the will of others, and the will of society as a whole. In order to prevent this development, many physicians hold the opinion that prenatal diagnosis and abortion can only be justified as long as the child is not viable. It is, however, dubitable whether this attitude is a sufficient stronghold against the rapidly increasing social pressure, in combination with international, partly even legally warranted tendencies, to prevent the birth of people with a disease or a handicap by all possible means and without time limits. Without unambiguous legal measures, such tendencies can hardly be successfully halted.

5. MORAL CONSIDERATIONS

The numerous moral issues surrounding prenatal diagnosis that we mentioned above, cannot be addressed exhaustively. We will have to confine ourselves to the two most essential moral notions which are affected by the new methods of genetic testing and prenatal medicine.

5.1. "Unworthy" Life?

The foremost moral complexity surrounding genetic counselling and prenatal diagnosis is not the aborting of diseased human lives, but the discussion about what establishes "worthy" and "unworthy" life that follows from these methods. Genetic testing and prenatal diagnosis undeniably necessitate that we make judgments about the value of life of non-healthy children. To be sure, we can confine the right to make such judgments to parents and to parents only. But these, of course, will have to make their judgments in the context of the society which surrounds them, in which judgments about the value of the lives of *other* persons become increasingly accepted. Many persons hold the opinion that the dignity and the value of a human life are rooted in, and indicated by empirically observable characteristics. According to some empiristic philosophers, someone can be seen as a human being if and only if he has a number of empirically observable qualities such as freedom, self-conscience, conscious interests, and the like.[16] Human personhood and its corresponding dignity are seen as identical to these empirical qualities, not to life as such. So if these qualities have not reached a certain stage of development, life does not bear the dignity of a human person. Likewise, life can loose its dignity as a consequence of diseases and decline. Humans loose the right to be respected and treated as persons. Ending such a life is not the killing of a person, and can therefore not be classified as wrong.

The crucial error of all those who advocate late abortions and early euthanasia is that they conceive dignity and value of life in terms of empirically observable qualities that are not given with life itself, and which can be destroyed as a consequence of diseases or handicaps. Such an empiristic conception of persons and personal value actively challenges us to make judgments about the value of life.

In a christian view, the dignity of being a human being and a person is not grounded in empirically knowable qualities, but in the fact that God created humans in his image and destined them to be in everlasting communion with himself.[17] This destination cannot be made undone, not even when physical, psychological or mental distortions keep a person from pursuing this destination. Someone is a human person because of what God did to him and for him. Human dignity is therefore a "transcendent" quality, which God has appointed at every moment in life (i.e., organic life) until death, and which remains. It cannot be lost, however damaged body and mind — in other words, the empirical personality — may have become. We have the duty to respect and act in accordance with this unalienable and, because God wanted it to live, inviolable human dignity.

Only if we — like in empiristic and partly even idealistic philosophy — identify person and personality, the decay of the latter warrants us to conclude that we can, under some given circumstances, no longer speak of a life that has full human dignity and value. Such a conclusion about the value of human life implies a total, and therefore deadly form of human determination over one's own life and the lives of others, which does not properly belong to any human individual, nor to society as a whole. Humans don't have the liberty to make judgments about the value of life, nor to attribute or to deny someone human dignity. Instead, we are called to acknowledge and affirm human dignity and value as given with life itself, and to respect and treat humans accordingly. This asks for the development of an ethos of care as outlined previously.

In prosperous and liberal western societies, there is no longer unanimity as to what establishes the dignity of human life and what undergirds the right to life and care. In my opinion, this might just be the ultimate consequence of the secularization of our worldview and our life-style, and of the refusal to accept a religiously based anthropology alike. When we no longer accept that people with a handicap (but not the handicap itself) are created by God just like any other, "healthy" human being, destined to reflect his image and intended to live in eternal fullness, we end up with a horizontal ideology without prospects for a restoration of our earthly lives. It is not surprising that such a constellation allows us to make judgments about "unworthy" human life: what is the meaning of a life when it lacks, alongside with all other, more or less "healthy" human beings, the promise of perfection in a hereafter, and when it consequently fails to see the uniqueness of this earthly life which God so loves?

5.2. Endurance and Solidarity with the Weak

Those in our societies who perform the often difficult task of caring for people with a handicap or a disease — parents, relatives, health care professionals —, need to have clarity about what exactly establishes the dignity, and what motivates the right to life and care of those they care for. This clarity provides, in turn, the appreciation which corresponds to the complexity of their vocations. Only in this manner, can a society grant the weakest of its members their proper care and concern. There is a definite risk that new medical methods to prevent the birth of diseased human lives will increasingly lead to doubts as to the right of unborn and born, handicapped, and chronically ill human beings. As the ethos of care for these people erodes, there is a risk that the concern for, and care of the "incurable" become seen as a "useless", "meaningless", and socially "counterproductive" activity, a pointless waste of personal and financial resources. In the long run, this will undermine the right to life and to a dignified care for all those persons, who — despite increasingly perfect prevention and therapy — have been born with handicaps, or who, in the course of their lives, have become incurably ill, severely handicapped, or care-dependent as a consequence of diseases or accidents.[18]

In classical civilization the glorification of the autonomous, mentally superior person (philosopher), and of the youthfully vital person (athlete), was already one of the main causes for the almost total failure of any ethos of compassion and of care for the weakest members of the community. Those who were "incurable", those who were "wronged" in body, mind, and spirit, were selected and expelled. Against this ethics of autonomy and strength, the christian church presented an explicitly anti-selectionist ethos of compassion, solidarity with, and care for the weakest members of the community. A view of man which leaves no room for incurability, illnesses, dependence, and decline of the human personality, and which is only interested in the highest mental, spiritual, and physical accomplishments — i.e., only in the strong and their happiness —, is a threat to the lives of the weakest members of the community. It expels any memory of "unhappy" and "unworthy" lives out of its midst and it is incapable of coping with suffering in any other way than by removing it by technical or "social-technical" means, if necessary even by denying suffering persons the necessary care.

Along with the growing technical possibilities of fighting and abandoning diseases and handicaps, Western societies are becoming increasingly incompetent of coming to terms with suffering, other than by these technical means. The humanity of a society, however, does not consist in its capacity to remove human suffering by medical- and social-technical means — e.g., through "euthanasia" —, but rather in the way it treats all those who are incurably ill, disabled, or otherwise in need of continuous care and concern. What counts, is its capacity to provide empathy and care to all those, who are seemingly or even effectively useless to the happiness of the majority of people but who, despite all this, inspire to a deeper understanding of what establishes true success and meaning in life.

Success in life not only comprises experiences of happiness, but also — as a necessary counterpart — the capacity to suffer and sympathy with those who suffer, without whom we will never be able to grasp the full reality of life. What at first sight seems to hinder our life happiness, could well prove to be a road towards success and happiness in a deeper sense. Respect for human dignity — especially of the incurable and of those who need continuous care — is just as valuable, if not more valuable, as health and a life without suffering. When the "urge for health" tends to develop into a threat to the dignity of and the care for the weakest members of a society, we should even consider to refrain from making therapeutical progress. If that is needed in order to safeguard the human dignity and the human rights of these people, it is well worth the sacrifice.[19]

NOTES

1 U. Eibach, *Liebe, Glück und Partnerschaft: Sexualität und Familie im Wertewandel* (Love, Happiness, and Partnership: Sexuality and Family in Changing Values). Wuppertal: Brockhaus, 1996, pp. 19ff.

2 Referring to Nazi-Germany may be offensive to some. On some occasions, however, such a comparison should be made. I do believe that the past may teach us some necessary, though bitter lessons. It may help to point to two circumstances here. First, making a comparison does *not* imply any allegations as to the intentions of anyone involved. Secondly, however, it should be noted that a considerable number of those who contributed to the developments in Nazi-Germany were not aware of the terrible consequences which their thinking was about to have.

3 U. Eibach, *Medizin und Menschenwürde. Ethische Probleme in der Medizin aus christlicher Sicht.* (Medicine and Human Dignity: Moral Problems in Medicine from a Christian Perspective). Wuppertal: Brockhaus, 1997[5], pp. 270 ff.

4 K. Binding and A. Hoche, *Die Freigabe der Vernichtung lebensunwerten Lebens: Ihr Masz und ihre Form* (The Allowance to Destroy Unworthy Life: Its Extent and Form). Leipzig: Felix Meiner, 1920.

5 Cf. W. Wolfensberger, *The New Genocide of Handicapped an Afflicted People.* Syracuse: Institute for Human Service Planning, Leadership and Change Agentry, 1987; B. Richarz, *Heilen, Pflegen, Töten* (Healing, Caring, Killing), Göttingen: Vandenhoeck 1987, pp. 200 ff.; K. Nowak, *"Euthanasie" und Sterilisierung im "Dritten Reich"* ("Euthanasia" and Sterilisation in the Third Reich). Göttingen: Vandenhoeck 1984; H.-W. Schmuhl, *Rassenhygiene, Nationalsozialismus, Euthanasie. Von der Verhütung zur Vernichtung "lebensunwerten Lebens"* (Racial Hygiene, National-Socialism, Euthanasia: From Prevention to Destruction of "Unworthy Life"). Göttingen: 1987.

6 V. von Weizsäcker, *Euthanasie und Menschenversuche* (Euthanasia and Experiments on Humans). *Psyche Folge 1.* Heidelberg: Schneider 1947, pp. 15 ff.

7 Cf. the Bible: Paul's letter to the Romans in Romans 8:18ff.

8 Cf. J.C. Tronto, *Moral Boundaries: A Political Argument for an Ethic of Care.* New York/ London: Routledge, 1993. See also the contributions of Theo A. Boer and Hans Reinders in this volume (chapters 4 and 5).

9 U. Eibach, "Vom Paternalismus zur Autonomie des Patienten?" (From Paternalism to Patient Autonomy?), *Zeitschrift für medizinische Ethik* 43 (1997), no. 2.

10 Cf. the Statement of the German Society for Human Genetics, *Zeitschrift für medizinische Ethik* 42 (1996), pp. 326 ff.

11 U. Eibach, *Gentechnik: der Griff nach dem Leben* (Genetic Technique: Seizing Life). Wuppertal: Brockhaus, 1988, pp. 139ff.

12 U. Eibach, "Ökonomische Grenzen des Gesundheitswesens und die Fürsorge für unheilbare und schwerstpflegebedürftige Menschen" (Economic Limits in Health Care and the Care of Incurable and People with Heavy Care Needs), *Kerygma und Dogma*, vol. 43 (1997), pp. 202ff.

13 H. Kuhse and P. Singer, *Should the Baby Live? The Problem of Handicapped Infants*. Oxford: Oxford University Press, 1985.

14 German Constitution, Section 2, subsection 3: "No one's rights may be infringed because of his handicap." Abortion on the basis of a handicap is seen as one such infringement. Hence, selective abortion can only take place on the basis of an assumed "unbearable burden" of the mother. See also U. Eibach, *Sterbehilfe: Tötung aus Mitleid? Euthanasie und "lebensunwertes" Leben* (Assisted Dying: Killing out of Compassion? Euthanasia and "Unworthy" Life). Wuppertal: Brockhaus 1998, pp. 164-170.

15 In November, 1998, the Federal Association of Physicians in Germany issued a recommendation not to do any abortions or to let fetuses die when they are already viable. To what extent this recommendation is respected, remains unclear. There are indications that in some instances, doctors now decide to terminate the life of the viable child while still in the womb shortly before it is born. For many of those who are involved in this process, killing the fetus in the womb is emotionally more burdensome than letting the fetus die by denying it care.

16 For this debate, cf. A. Peacoke, G. Gillet (eds.), *Persons and Personality*. Oxford: Oxford University Press 1987; K. Bayertz (ed.), *Sanctity of Life and Human Dignity*. Dordrecht: Kluwer 1996; U. Eibach, *Sterbehilfe* (1998), pp. 60ff.

17 Eibach, *Medizin und Menschenwürde* 1993, pp. 83ff. Evangelische Kirche in Deutschland (Protestant Church in Germany), a.o.: *Gott ist ein Freund des Lebens* (God is a Friend of Life). Gütersloh: Gerd Mohn 1989, pp. 46ff.

18 Cf. note 13.

19 Cf. note 9 and Eibach, *Sterbehilfe: Tötung aus Mitleid?* (1998), pp 67ff., 148ff.

DINY VAN BRUGGEN

CHAPTER 8

MEANINGFULNESS AND MEANINGLESSNESS IN NEONATOLOGY

1. THE UNUSUAL LIFE OF BABY K.

In the *Lancet* of October 1993, a case study was presented on the life of Baby K., a baby girl born with anencephaly.[1] Before birth the baby was already diagnosed with this very serious congenital birth defect. In babies with anencephaly the vault of the skull is absent, and though the brainstem is present, the cerebral cortex is rudimentary or absent. In the case of Baby K. it meant that she had reflex actions like respiration and reflex actions to touch and sound, but she never would gain consciousness. There is no cure for this disorder. Without medical interventions these children die within days to weeks after birth, (though exceptions have been described). When Baby K. was born, she did not breathe. She was put on artificial ventilation, awaiting . . . who knows? The mother insisted on continued intensive care and refused to give permission for a do-not-resuscitate order. The doctors wanted to limit their interventions to comfort care or to care-for-the-dying and viewed the intensive treatment as not appropriate. The case was dealt with in court and the judge decided that the intensive treatment had to be continued. The physicians were furious: "Next, we'll have to give her [this child without cerebral cortex] an artificial kidney or perform a liver or heart transplant."

The physicians and the mother each had their reasons which, taken on their own, all were hard to contradict. Baby K. lived to the age of two and a half years. Years full of disputes, court cases, hurt mother's feelings, ignored father's input and unrest in society. She died after another resuscitation attempt, which this time did not succeed.[2] The life of Baby K. is just one example of the seemingly unsolvable questions that can arise concerning medical technical interventions in the area of life and death and in dealing with severe handicaps. It can easily be supplemented with many more examples from the NICU's (neonatal intensive care units), where these sick newborns are being treated. It leads us to considering very basic questions regarding decisions, taken in medical treatments.

Joop Stolk, Theo A. Boer & Ruth Seldenrijk (eds.). Meaningful Care, 113—125

2. THE UNUSUAL DYING OF BABY K.

The case of (non)treatment of Baby K. was reviewed in many articles. One of them starts with the most basic question: "Are anencephalic newborns dead or alive?"[3] The answer goes back to the question: What constitutes a living person? Does the life of a person start at the conception or afterwards? Which criteria — for example to be able to gain consciousness — are critical? How do we define death and brain-death? Some authors call anencephalic children "babies with imminent death," but this description could need revision after a publication in which unexpected survival of two such infants to an age of respectively 7 and 10 months was described.[4]

These questions are of utmost importance and have become even more relevant in the discussions on taking out organs for transplantation. But dealing with them exceeds the scope of this chapter.

In the case of Baby K. the diagnosis was made before birth and the mother was offered the option of induced abortion. She refused, arguing: "each life is given by God and only He can take it". After birth the baby did not breathe but since the mother requested full life support for her child, the baby was put on artificial ventilation. The mother knew that the child never would gain consciousness, but her belief that God can do miracles made her insist on her requests. The father had a different opinion. His preference was to withdraw medical treatment and to allow the child to die. His request was not granted, since he was not wed to the mother and was not very attached to the child.

After one month the baby was transferred to a nursing home, but on the condition that she would be re-admitted to intensive care in case her condition deteriorated. She was resuscitated several times in intensive care. She even got a tracheotomy (artificial opening in the airway) to facilitate future artificial ventilation, if needed. Although the doctors preferred to withdraw treatment, the pressure on them continued. The case was dealt with in several court cases and each time the verdict was to continue aggressive medical treatment.

The mother had strong arguments for her case. She referred to "the right of parents to make medical treatment decisions for their minor children. This refers to the concern for the constitutional principles of family autonomy."[5] She also seemed to have the Rehabilitation Act on her side. Refusing emergency treatment to a baby, simply because of the degree of the handicap of the baby is unacceptable discrimination under the Act.[6] Other authors even stated that the doctor always has to provide the requested life-saving treatment, since non-physicians are not licensed to life-prolonging techniques. Therefore the doctor, in his monopoly position, should always follow the patient's request, even if it seems to him to be an intolerable deviation from the standard care.[7] The physicians could not live with this consumer-concept of health care. It does not take into account their professional input and their duty to treat according to nationally agreed upon standards. And doctors cannot be pressed to give treatment that is futile. The most clear example of this is: they cannot be pressed to resuscitate a person, whom they consider to be dead.

In the USA, another law played an important role in this discussion. In order to prevent private hospitals from sending away poor people who need emergency treatment, there is a law that all patients in a hospital should always receive emergency treatment. But applied in this case the law was used in a sense that all patients, even dying patients, for whom treatment is futile, should be resuscitated, if this is the wish of the relatives.

3. MEANINGFUL: LIFE OR ACTIONS

The decision to treat or not-to-treat Baby K. has many more aspects than strictly medical technical ones. We have already seen some consequences resulting from our views regarding being a person, handicaps, the parents-child relationship and the doctor-patient relationship. But there is still more. An ethicist concluded: "We are talking here about the value of life without consciousness. The answer is philosophically or religiously determined".[8] If his conclusion is correct, there is not much left to say for a practising physician.

Nevertheless, the story of Baby K. is the starting point of this chapter. The ethicist was right: the basic question about the meaning of this life — or, in this case, the meaning of the life of an anencephalic child — cannot be answered by medical sciences. The same is true for the question whether this human life has enough dignity or value. These questions are not medical at heart, but religious or philosophical. On the other hand, discussions about meaningfulness or meaninglessness are also the doctor's business, but in another, more restricted sense: he assesses whether certain forms of *care* are meaningful, not whether the *life of a person with a handicap* is meaningful. Our overview of the life of Baby K. leaves us with the question: is artificial ventilation of an anencephalic child a meaningful medical treatment? And this case study could easily be extended to many more similar cases from the NICU's. Though the mother and the doctors each had plausible arguments, they never were able to agree on the type of treatment. This chapter will deal with these problems in more detail, with the main question: how can you decide what is meaningful medical care?

4. MEDICAL INTERVENTION

Before we talk about meaningful medical care, we must first define the meaning of "medical care" . Medical care has been defined for centuries as: to heal the sick, and when this is not possible, to ease the suffering. Later, another objective was added: when possible, to prevent illness. In the meantime, the understanding of what "health" meant was greatly stretched. From being primarily focused on physical wellbeing, the definition of health became: a state of physical, psychological, and spiritual wellbeing. This concept was embraced internationally at the Alma Ata conference (1978).[9] Expectations were high. The creed of Alma Ata was: health for all by the year 2000.[10]

There has been improvement in the area of health care in western countries. Yet, areas remain for which modern medicine has few answers.[11] In neonatology there have also been great advances, but after starting life in the intensive care unit, some children survived only to the cost of having very serious handicaps.

Alongside with these developments, a new element was introduced in the last decade. For some physicians, medical care could even comprise the termination of a life: "if needed, end the life of the patient in order to make an end to the suffering . . ."[12] Sometimes, such life-terminating actions are even called "secondary prevention".[13] Even though, internationally, this last development in medical practice has not been accepted by all, it has become relatively broadly accepted in the Netherlands, albeit not without debate. This has tremendous consequences. The question whether terminating a life can be a medical intervention (or "completion of a medical intervention") may have an impact on decisions that are made regarding treatments. A decision to walk down a particular (medical) path strongly depends on the possibilities at the end of the way. If the termination of life is one of the alternatives, it is not impossible that this may discourage physicians from trying to find other solutions.

5. MEANINGFUL MEDICAL CARE

Before proceeding, we need to define what *meaningful medical care* is. I would describe it as "a medical intervention that is *medically* beneficial". Medical benefit often is more narrowly described in terms of "effective treatment" and "greater benefits than risks". Is treatment not effective, or if it harms the patient in a disproportionate way, i.e., brings about more risks than benefits, we would be better off calling it *mal*-treatment. We could go one step further and define medical care meaningful if and only if "the situation is better for the patient after the intervention than before it." In this last option, medical care in which the patient is *not* better off, may be regarded as meaningless. Note: the point of measurement is not the effectiveness of the intervention in an isolated, medical sense, but the effect it has on the well-being of the patient!

In order to weigh and measure whether an intervention leads to an improvement or a deterioration in the patient's condition, we must develop a good measurement tool. I am reminded of a proud surgeon, who managed to straighten a rigidly bent finger after four surgeries, although the finger remained rigid. Considering the fact that the patient was a typist, she now really was disabled. In spite of some fine medical-technical results, the medical intervention was a failure. When determining the benefit of an intervention, we therefore must take into account the associated costs and burdens. If, for instance, a medical treatment is reasonably successful, but the patient ends up with lasting and persistent pain which is worse after the intervention than beforehand, the intervention was in this sense, medically meaningless.

Concluding that an intervention is medically meaningless, however, does not imply the option to end the life of someone with a handicap on the assumption that "death would be better for this person than a damaged life." For such decisions, physicians have no measuring tools.[14] Moreover, the deliberate and active termination of the life of a human being falls in a totally different moral category in comparison to decisions to stop treatment.

Many early publications describe that doctors treated patients with all available means, not regarding the meaningfulness of the action. I doubt this.[15] In those days there were many more hopeless situations with untreatable diseases than nowadays. Think of the position of lepers. Their life was more unbearable and without prospect than life for most patients today. Nevertheless nobody considered euthanasia. Their desperate situation ended by promoting better care and acceptance and later by the discovery of a cure by effective drugs. This attitude did not change till the middle of this century.[16] A possible exception, it may be said, was the treatment of patients with rabies in a terminal phase. When watching them suffer became unbearable, these patients were sometimes suffocated. This suffocation was more an action of despair, however, than a part of the medical treatment.[17]

The prospects for treatment and palliative care have greatly increased in the past decades, first with better patient care, and later with the availability of more effective medications. Notwithstanding the enhancements of medical treatment in the past decades, we witness an increasing willingness to put an end to human lives by means of active medical intervention.

In summary: meaningful medical care is medically-technically effective, it is beneficial for the patient, and it is proportional. In the field of neonatology, it is often hard to decide if a treatment fulfills all criteria of meaningfulness. The story of Baby K.'s artificial respiration is an example of the complexity of this issue. Was the phycisian's intervention effective, was it beneficial, was it proportional? Even if we assume that all this is the case, treatment in other cases may be more problematic to choose. With an anencephalic child, the end result is relatively predictable, but in many other cases, there are more uncertainties. When, e.g., you start treating an infant born at 25 weeks gestation, you can say little about the outcome for this child. Perhaps treatment will bring about something good, perhaps not. The uncertainties are vast.

6. POLICY DEVELOPMENTS IN NEONATOLOGY

Notwithstanding the complexity of the subject-matter, several attempts have been made to formulate some form of policy in neonatology. In 1990, a report of the Royal Dutch Association of Medicine appeared, entitled: *Life-terminating Interventions with Incompetent Patients, Part 1: Severely Defective Newborns.*[18] Although many valuable points are raised, the report suggests a worrisome procedure. With each child, a ruler of positive and negative properties is applied. If the net-results are insufficient, the report argues, the physician should have the option to end the child's life.

A subsequent report was issued in 1992 by the Dutch Association for Paediatrics: *To Act or Not to Act: Limits of Medical Care in Neonatology.*[19] This report deserves more praise: the complicated area with which it deals, is carefully and systematically mapped out, and the treatment options are clearly defined. The report first identifies four options:

- one can decide to treat newborns with the use of all available means;
- one can decide to intervene with all means, but only as long as there are no complications or until a certain limit has been reached;

- one can decide to stop all life support, while continuing to use an incubator and tube-feed as usual;
- in certain instances, one can decide to cease all medical interventions, and to ease the dying process by medicating.

As to these alternatives, none of the paediatricians had objections to the report; the concepts and distinctions were appreciated for the clarity they give when working in a team-context. Yet, opinions differed on the two subsequent options: accelerating the dying process in order to prevent an inhumanely difficult death, and the purposeful termination of life in case of emergency.

In the Netherlands, these two latter options have been put into practice and tried in court. In 1993, a physician was acquitted after ending the life of a child with bifid spine and other complications.[20] In 1995, a physician was acquitted after terminating the life of a child with trisomy 13.[21] In 1996, this food for thought was belabored further during a symposium in Utrecht: *On the Verge of Life and Death.*[22] At the conference, a panel of physicians and ethicists was requested to assess whether a decision for life-termination is justified as the completion of a medical intervention. Opinions at the conference did not differ in regards to whether and when one should forego instituting or extending a meaningless intervention. Even here, however, there were differences of opinion whether or not life-terminating actions should be allowed in such instances.[23] One way or the other, the latter option now has become part of the political discussion in the Netherlands, with an increasing focus on the quality of life. In this discussion, it has now been decided that committees will be established which will judge interventions surrounding the end of life. Concerning the life of people with a handicap *before* birth, however, the verdict has long been made. It has become a fairly common practice for physicians and parents to assume that, because of his handicap, the unborn child would be better off not living. In the Netherlands, more than half of all children with Down Syndrome are diagnosed before they are born, and made to die by means of a selective abortion.[24] When a child with Down Syndrome is born, the health care system is often blamed for its poor preventive medicine; sometimes, the parents are deemed to be "at fault".[25]

After the birth, however, there is a different picture. New surgical techniques and early intervention programs have greatly improved the prognosis of these children.[26] In related discussions, the term, "quality of life" is used with increasing frequency.

7. QUALITY OF LIFE

In the earlier mentioned report *To Act or Not to Act* of the Dutch Association for Paediatrics in the Netherlands, quality of life is described on the basis of the following characteristics:

- communication possibilities
- degree of suffering
- level of independence
- dependence on the medical circuit
- life expectancy

These are important criteria. They are useful in describing a child's medical and biological potential — and his limitations. Life, however, is more than its biological potential. These criteria may serve as guidelines for physicians and other health care professionals to direct the treatment according to the specific needs of the child. If, for example, we know that a child never will be able to walk, there is less need to worry about his foot deviation. Yet, such considerations should never become a criteria for deciding if the person should die. After all, they don't speak of the ultimate quality of his life, nor of the "meaning" of his life.

As a reaction to this report, the Dutch Federation of Parent Associations (FVO) published the brochure, *Equal Opportunities*.[27] The brochure wastes no words: "Handicaps should never be a reason to forego a treatment." This reaction, however understandable, is in my opinion too black and white. A handicap could actually be the reason why a medical treatment could be of no effect, because of its proportionality, or because this particular patient wouldn't medically benefit from the treatment. The decision becomes especially difficult when the chance for a positive result is unsure,[28] or when there is a statistic chance that some children will benefit, whereas many others will suffer additionally. Let us imagine a group of 100 children: is it permitted to allow 99 of them to suffer for the benefit of the one that you could save? This is a matter of statistics and calculating the odds. How can this take place?

8. STATISTICS AND CALCULATING THE ODDS

Lately, much follow-up research has been performed with children in NICU's (Neonatal Intensive Care Units) and paediatric surgical ICU's. Much is already known about percentages and odds.[29] But statistics say nothing about the chances of the individual child. It could well be that a certain treatment, which has proved to be effective and beneficial to some, will put additional suffering on others. It is not uncommon that parents get the impression that "the medical powers bouldered over" their child.[30] An example: since the seventies, children with bifid spine were treated according to the criteria of Lorber in several medical centers.[31] Only the children with the best odds were operated on. As it is extremely difficult to create good selection criteria for corrective surgery, even the Lorber-criteria received criticism.[32] But what is the alternative? In my opinion, it is therefore also wrong not to try.

To take another example: what should one do with a child who is born with a shaky start at 25 weeks gestation? If we offer the maximum medical-technical treatment available, there is a chance that he will survive. There will, however, be a risk for blindness, intracranial bleeding, and pulmonary problems. Thus, some physicians will not treat: in their eyes, the possibility of adding to the infant's suffering is too great. Others will — generally — treat; they figure that the odds for a positive result are sufficiently good. Yet others judge whether the child fulfills a number of criteria. Only then will they begin the intensive treatment.

9. "CHANCE TREATMENT": THE HUNTER'S DILEMMA

Setting "criteria for treatment" has its pros and cons. If one were to decide that the artificial ventilation of infants born before 24 weeks gestation would bring on too much suffering for too many of these infants, one could decide not to intervene at all. They would all die. Even that one strong infant, that could have made it. To be able to save this one child, without adding suffering to the others, it is argued that all infants should be given a "chance treatment".

Before we delve into this subject, let us consider this example from the field of ethics. A hunter sees something moving in the woods. Is it a deer? Or could it be a human person? Even if the chance of it being a person is just 1%, the hunter will decide not to shoot. He will let the deer go, rather than risking the death of a human.

About the hunter's decision to let the deer go, there will probably not be much argument. Let us, however, imagine a more complicated situation. The hunter sees something moving in the bushes. As he looks closer, he perceives a man being attacked by a lion. The hunter, of course, wants to save the man, but will he be able to shoot the lion and only the lion? If he succeeds in shooting the lion only, the hunter will be considered a hero. But if he accidentally kills or wounds the man, the evaluation of his decision to shoot will probably be less positive.

The hunters in these situations have a choice. They will have to decide based on an assessment of their skills and of the odds. The skilled hunter shoots, as he expects to be able to hit the lion without wounding the man. His less skilled colleague would rather wait. Maybe the man will be able to escape without help.

This all changes if the following policy is introduced: if the result of his action is disappointing, a hunter is allowed to kill the man. Acting on this policy, the hunters shoot each time. As a result of this, they save many lives. Of the survivors, none is wounded because if this test-shot, this "chance treatment", has wounded a man, he may, after all, still be killed. In other words: there are only healthy survivors. One could imagine that some heated discussions would ensue about the conditions under which the hunter would be allowed to kill the wounded man.

To be sure, in current-day medical practice, we don't work with lions. Yet, there are comparable situations: a man (patient), a lion (disease), and a rescue-operation (treatment) which could cause considerable damage to the patient. Physicians must consider the pros and cons, and must take great risks. Sometimes, the risk is considered to be too great. The physician would not treat a child of this category, because he knows that one case of success will, statistically, cause other children to suffer more intensely. In a way, therefore, the physician is powerless in saving this child, because the price is too high when viewed in the larger context. This would be the option I would choose; a physician will have to acknowledge his *powerlessness* in cases similar to this, and should refrain from undertaking interventions if the risks are too high. If one's medical power does not deliver positive results, one ought to acknowledge his powerlessness rather than covering it up by usurping even more power and by pretending to be all-powerful.

In current day medicine, the physician often opts for another alternative: to gain and exert more and more power, and to strive for the highest possible power: power over the life of the patient, even when the results of the treatment may turn out to be disappointing. To many in neonatology, this seems an attractive option. If the physician has that power, he can always start a "chance treatment". Yet, this attractive phrase, "chance treatment" fails to describe the *real* situation. With a "chance treatment," it is not the treatment, but the person's *life* that gets a chance. The patient is given a chance, but afterwards does have to fulfill certain criteria. If he fails to do so, life-terminating actions are considered.

An example is the story of Nora and Willy, who were both born much too early.[33] Nora survives because of an intervention. She is now a radiant one year old. In Willy's case, however, everything goes wrong. After three weeks, he is able to breathe on his own, but already has severe brain damage. The doctors and the parents face a dilemma. Willy was given a chance, but not with the intention to keep him alive in order to let him suffer for years. As Willy's life did not fit the operative criteria for quality, his life was ended.

10. PARENT SUPPORT

The parent's part in all this is described in more detail in chapters one, two, and nine. Meaningful medical care of the newborn is only possible with parent involvement. Having a child with a handicap or a very premature or immature child can be described as a double process. The child you expected did not arrive. You now have to "bury" all your expectations. And then there is that other child, as if "from a different nest".[34] We don't know what to think about its defects. And we may be terribly worried about its future.[35]

As a consequence, a period of great ambivalence in the relationship of the parents and their child follows. Even physicians often don't know what to do during this period. Some try to prevent parents from bonding with their child. The child is pictured as a product, with whom we can't develop a relationship. The reaction of many parents is to want to escape. They want their child to die. Only few dare to voice this desire or bring it to consciousness. It is important to pay attention to these issues directly after birth, such as in the labour and delivery unit, or even before birth. Each set of parents will react differently, depending on their own experiences. Even their needs and questions will change with time.[36]

In the case of a congenital defect, many parents have to face additional complexities. On the basis of their experience, physicians can sometimes predict that a child belonging to a certain category of patients has a poor life expectancy. A child isn't a statistic however, and has a life of his own. In meetings with the parents, it is important to bring up that the child could die shortly, but that it could also stay alive for some (limited amount of) time. If one begins anticipating the death too soon, it seems to come too slowly and the task of supporting the parents may become more difficult than is necessary.

Therapeutic interventions should be within proportion. For a dying child, many curative, therapeutic interventions might be disproportional. One ought to now fully attend to the palliative side of care, to relieving the suffering. This leaves many possibilities. Because the life expectancy is limited, many side effects can be seen in a different light. At the end of the day, it is not that important whether this child dies with a good blood-sugar level, an undamaged liver, or a good EEG. For a dying child, a stay in the intensive care unit is usually contraindicated, as his or her death is not only expected, but also unavoidable. If the child dies while receiving good pain management, the child has been cared for well.

Supporting the parents is of paramount importance in the days, weeks, or months surrounding the unequal battle for the child. It may be an important time for creating some precious memories, memories which will be remembered for the rest of the parents' lives. Pictures of parents with the child (in which defects are covered or hidden), presents of brothers or sisters, and other little touches will create special memories of this little sibling, who had been looked forward to so much, but who will only stay so briefly. An additional way of supporting the parents is to refer them to parent associations of the handicapped, where they might find other parents with similar experiences.

11. CONCLUSION

To perform medically meaningful actions means that they are effective, have medical benefit, and are proportional. Our primary consideration should not be the choice between life and or death; rather, the focus should be on the question whether an intervention offers anything positive. For this, we especially look at life expectancy, relieving of suffering, and level of functioning. The categories listed in the report of the Dutch Association for Paediatrics are of great value herein.

If we treat (medically) meaningfully, Baby K., the child with anencephaly to whom we referred in the beginning of this chapter, would possibly have lived only a few days. With a little hat to cover the large head wound, and many kisses from his parents in farewell. In my opinion, medical treatments were out of proportion in this case. Nora, the very premature infant, would still be alive, thankful for all the great developments in neonatology. Willy might also still be alive, with serious brain damage. Despite the disappointing results of the medical intervention, however, there is no reason to end his life. He is a continuous reminder of the tensions that are present in choosing whether to treat or not.

We will always do everything in our power to prevent a handicap. Each person with a handicap will wish along with us for handicaps to disappear as much as possible. We are, however, not justified in doing this by removing people with a handicap.

The question remains: what is the meaning of life with a handicap? Stated differently: what is the meaning of Willy's life? Everyone has their own answer to this question. I have my own individual answer, as do most parents of children with a handicap. The answers are beyond the purpose of this chapter, and some of them may be found elsewhere in this book. It is my conviction that our answers should not play that big a role: it is too risky to make the life of a random individual dependent on the fact whether another person, such as the physician, considers his life meaningful. If this were the case, the physician would be omnipotent.

NOTES

1 M. McCarthy, "Anencephalic baby's right to life?", *The Lancet*, vol. 342, October 9, (1993), p. 919.
2 J. Paris, "Guidelines on the Care of Anencephalic Infants: a Response to Baby K", *Journal of Perinatology*, vol. 15, no. 4, 1995, p. 318-324.
3 S. Fry-Revere, "Anencephalic newborns: legal and ethical comments regarding the matter of baby 'K'", *Paediatric Nursing*, vol. 20, no. 3 (May-June 1994), pp. 283-6.
4 G. McAbee *et al.*, "Prolonged survival of two anencephalic infants", *American Journal of Perinatology*, vol. 10, no. 2 (March 1993), pp. 175-7.
5 See Paris (1995).
6 Fry-Revere (1994) p. 284.
7 See Paris (1995) p. 322.
8 See McCarthy (1993) p. 919.
9 World Health Organization, *Primary Health Care: Report of the International Conference on Primary Health Care.* Alma Ata, USSR, 1978.
10 In the meantime, the year 2000 approaches; health for everyone in this world is a distant concept. This goal was subsequently adjusted and narrowed down. "Health care for everyone" became "primary health care", which was further narrowed down to a few subjects, such as vaccinations. Now, close to 2000, the only big goal that remains is: worldwide eradication of polio. The outlook worldwide for neonatology is somber.
11 The most important of these are: living with chronic illnesses and handicaps, and the dying process.
12 B. Verschuren and C. Versluys, *Grenzen van medische behandeling bij pasgeborenen met een ernstige aandoening* (Limits of Medical Treatment of Newborns with Severe Conditions). Baarn: VSOP Publishers, no. 6.
13 "Until a few years ago, NTD prevention was only possible by means of prenatal research" (NTD = Neural Tube Defect). Later is stated, "this however is not true prevention". A.L. den Ouden *et al.*, "Prevalentie, klinisch beeld en prognose van neuraalbuisdefecten in Nederland" (Prevalence, Diagnosis, and Prognosis of Neural Tube Defects), *Nederlands Tijdschrift voor Geneeskunde*, Vol. 140, no 42 (1996), pp. 2092-4.
14 W.L.H. Smelt, H. Jochemsen, G. van Bruggen, and D.J. Bakker, "Een medisch ethisch commentaar" (Some Medical Ethical Comments), *Tijdschrift voor Geneeskunde en Ethiek,* Vol. 5, no. 1 (1995), pp.28-9.
15 He would have wanted to lengthen each human life at all costs, even if this brought along much suffering and a limited positive outcome. Undoubtedly, this happened at times. Yet, the physician used to know his own limits. If he had nothing to offer, he didn't bother the patient with medical treatments. Moreover, the hospitals carried more medical supplies than one had at home, such as oxygen. Yet, practically all the elderly would die at home, and not after a senseless stay in the intensive care unit of the hospital.
16 "Haeckel believed that numerous uncurably ill people were being kept alive artificially. As a result, the total number of patients in mental institutions in France would have increased by 30% over a period of 17 years. For that reason, Haeckel argues for the life termination of uncurably ill and seriously suffering patients, provided that the patient requests it, and that it be executed by a committee of physicians. Haeckel's arguments are: [...] the suffering of the patient and [...] the uselessness of staying alive." R.W.M. Croughs, "Euthanasie: een vergelijking van de huidige discussie in Nederland met de discussie in Duitsland vòòr 1933" ("Euthanasia: Comparing the Recent Dutch Discussion and the Discussion in Germany before 1933"), in: J. Stolk, *Gebroken wereld – zwakzinnigenzorg en de vraag naar euthanasie* (Broken World: Care of People with Mental Retardation and the Request for Euthanasia). Kampen: Kok Publishers, 1998.
17 From the diary of Jacob Bicker Raye: "May 30, 1751 [...] a child that was bitten by a rabid dog, and after being observed by many doctors was considered incurably rabid, was suffocated'. ...In my interpretation, this means that active euthanasia used to be considered permissible in the case of rabies, even indicated, and not practised with infrequency." G.A. Lindeboom, *Euthanasie in historisch perspectief* (Euthanasia: a Historical Overview). Amsterdam: Rodopi Publishers, 1978, pp. 23-4.
18 *Levensbeëindigend handelen bij wilsonbekwame patiënten. Deel I: zwaar-defecte pasgeborenen.* Utrecht: Koninklijke Nederlandsche Maatschappij tot Bevordering der Geneeskunst, 1990.

19 *Doen of laten? Grenzen van het medisch handelen in de neonatologie*. Utrecht: Dutch Association for Paediatrics, 1992.

20 See the following statement of the Court of Justice at Amsterdam, November 7, 1995: "witness D does not see any medical benefit in fighting the pain in such cases, and determines that in the given circumstances it was preferable to terminate the life of Rianne rather than managing the pain until the natural occurrence of death." "Expert E points out that... it would have been possible to treat the pain... but not medically beneficial... since death clearly was the planned outcome." "The judge determined that... treatment in the form of pain management was not beneficial." "Uitspraak van het gerechtshof te Amsterdam d.d. 7 november 1995" (Verdict of the Amsterdam Court), *Medisch Contact*, Vol. 51, no. 6 (1996), pp. 196-9.

21 Statement of the County Court at Groningen, November 13, 1995. "Uitspraak van de arrondissementsrechtbank te Groningen d.d. 13 november 1995", *Medisch Contact*, vol. 51, no 6. (1996), pp. 199-202.

22 T. van Willigenburg and W. Kuis (eds.), *Op de grens van leven en dood: afzien van behandelen en levensbeëindiging in de neonatologie* (On the Verge of Life and Death: Refraining from Treatment and Life Termination in Neonatology). Assen: Van Gorcum & Co. (1995).

23 Also see: G. van Bruggen, "Kinderartsen en gehandicapte baby's: de situatie anno 1996" (Paediatricians and Handicapped Babies: the Situation in 1996), in *Pro Vita Humana*, Vol. 3, no. 1 (1996), pp. 1-5.

24 Percentage of aborted cases in relation to total number of reported cases of Down's syndrome, the Northern Netherlands, 1994: of mothers in the age range 38-39 years: 75%; age range 40+ years: 100%; average of all age ranges: 55.6%. The abortions were induced around 17-18 weeks of gestation. Therefore, of the children with Down's syndrome in 1994, 55% did not live to see their expected birth-date thanks to prenatal diagnosis followed by a selective abortion. (International Clearinghouse for birth defects monitoring systems, a non-governmental organisation in official relations with the World Health Organisation, *Report 1995/96*, pp. 134-5).

25 Compare: E.E.E. van Wijck, B. Sikken, and M.J. Dekker, *Beeldvorming bij artsen over mensen met een verstandelijke handicap* (How Physicians See People with Mental Retardation). Groningen: Wetenschapswinkel Geneeskunde en Volksgezondheid, State University, 1995, p. 25.

26 Also see: *Het syndroom van Down, wat is optimale zorg?* (Down's Syndrome: what is Optimal Care?) Rotterdam: PAOG, in collaboration with Foundation for Down Syndrome Team Voorburg, 1996. The entire publication reflects the greatly improved care of children with Down's syndrome. Only the chapter, "The unborn child with Down's syndrome", paints a different picture. Here is only spoken of "diagnostic procedures", with considerable risks for the unborn child (0.3 – 1% chance of miscarriage) and a possible "intervention". During this period, an intervention consists of induced abortion: the termination of the life of the unborn child.

27 *Gelijke kansen. Medisch handelen rond pasgeborenen met een (verstandelijke) handicap* (Equal Opportunities: Medical Treatment of Newborns with Mental Retardation). Utrecht: FVO, 1993.

28 The FVO talks of the necessity to treat all newborns, since "it is basically impossible to make a concrete statement regarding the expected life outcome immediately after birth" (see FVO (1993) p. 11, note 24). This is true if one is talking about an individual. It is possible, however, to make such a statement about a total patient population.

29 D. Tibboel, *et al.*, "Grenzen aan de zorg; evaluatie van de besluitvorning rond het overlijden van 104 kinderen op een afdeling chirurgische Intensieve Zorg" (Limits of Care: Evaluating the Decisions around the Death of 104 Children in a Department of Surgical Intensive Care), *Nederlands Tijdschrift voor Geneeskunde,* Vol. 138, no. 19 (1994), pp. 953-8. M.J.K. de Kleine *et al.*, "Voortzetten of staken van levensverlengend handelen bij pasgeborenen: een onderzoek in 4 centra voor neonatale intensieve zorg" (Continuing or Withdrawal of Life Sustaining Treatment of Newborns: a Survey in Four Centers of Intensive Neonatal Care), *Nederlands Tijdschrift voor Geneeskunde*, Vol. 137, no. 10 (1993), pp. 496-500.

30 "The medical powers bouldered over her a couple of times. Thanks to them, she has to live this life." Comment of one of the parents in: J. Stolk and H. Kars, *Licht en schaduw: een onderzoek naar de zinervaring van ouders en groepsleiders in de zorg voor kinderen met een ernstige, meervoudige handicap* (Light and Shadow: a Survey of the Experiences of Meaning of Parents and Group Leaders in the Care of Children with Profound Multiple Handicaps). Amersfoort: Vereniging 's Heeren Loo, 1998, pp. 114-5.

31 J. Lorber, "Results of selective treatment of spina bifida cystica," *Archives of Disease in Childhood*, Vol. 56 (1981), pp. 822-30. Surgery would not be offered to the group with poor results. The group that was excluded from receiving surgical intervention would have a 50% chance of dying after the surgery, 30% would be severely handicapped, and 20% would only be motor-handicapped. Instead, they now all died. With this approach, the mortality rate of the group as a whole increased from 30-50% to 70%: more children died. But of the children that did receive surgical intervention, and of those that lived, a smaller percentage was seriously handicapped.

32 J.J. Rotteveel *et al.*, "Actieve levensbeëindiging bij pasgeborenen met spina bifida?" (Life Termination of Newborns with Bifid Spine?), *Nederlands Tijdschrift voor Geneeskunde*, Vol. 140, no. 14 (1996), pp. 799-803. J.J. Rotteveel reported that "in the dilemma of having respect for the human life and of the medical call to attempt to eradicate all factors leading to bio-medical accidents, there is, in our opinion, no place for active life termination. [. . .]" This is an area of tension within which it certainly will be appropriate, in certain cases, to discuss where the priority should lie. It is our hope that discussions take place within the profession in which a code of conduct could be created. This is more valuable than these trial cases. Also see: A.L. Staal-Schreinemachers *et al.*, "Toekomstperspectieven voor kinderen met spina bifida aperta" (Prospects for Children with Bifid Spine), *Nederlands Tijdschrift voor Geneeskunde*, Vol. 140, no. 24 (1996), pp. 1268-71.

33 Cited from reports in newspapers, in particular: *Nederlands Dagblad*, February 8, 1997.

34 "Mongoloid; this word was written on our hearts like a sentence; sometimes he seemed to me like a strange animal, having crawled out of a different nest." From: G. Jansen-Smit, "Ons godsgeschenk" (God's Gift to Us), in *Een hand die in de mijne past* (Poetry and Sayings about the World of People with Mental Retardation). Wezep: Bredewold Printers.

35 And, of course, other reactions of a psychosocial nature: the shock and shame felt by the parents when they find out their child is handicapped, the difficulty bonding with their child, and the reactions of their community (such as disappointed grandparents, or "how will I tell people at my work-place?").

36 "As the child gets older, the parents bond more with their child and find the thought of ending the life of their child more difficult" (p. 191). J. Stolk and A. van der Poel-van Vuuren, "Meningen van ouders over euthanasie bij hun ernstig gehandicapte kind" (Parents about Euthanasia of their Severely Handicapped Child), *Nederlands Tijdschrift voor Zwakzinnigenzorg*, no. 8 (1980), pp. 183-92.

JOOP STOLK AND HENK KARS

CHAPTER 9

PARENTS' VIEW ON THE PREVENTION OF HANDICAPS

1. INTRODUCTION

In chapter two, we reported on our research study about the experience of meaning of parents of a child with profound multiple handicaps. We limited ourselves to the first three research questions. In this chapter, we will address the fourth research question: has the way in which others value the life of children with profound multiple handicaps influenced the experience of meaning of the parents? If so, how? Given the complex nature of the interplay between the individual and his environment, we decided to limit ourselves to the question whether, and if so, how the discussion in society about the prevention of handicaps has influenced parents' experiences of meaning. We will start to focus on developments in diagnostic methods (section 2), the discussion about abortion with prenatally diagnosed handicaps (section 3), and the selective non-treatment of newborn children with profound multiple handicaps (section 4). After that, we will more specifically address the question whether, and, if so, how, society's discussion on the prevention of handicaps has influenced the experience of meaning of the parents (section 5).

2. DEVELOPMENTS IN DIAGNOSTIC METHODS

The conversation about the "prevention of handicaps" was started by means of a question that was usually framed as follows: "we have now come to the next subject. This is related to developments in the medical sciences, which have opened up many possibilities for the early diagnosis of a handicap. This might be in the form of genetic testing, before pregnancy is even considered. Another form would be an amniocentesis during the pregnancy. The test results might lead to the prevention of the birth of a child with a handicap, possibly by means of an abortion. What is your take on these developments?"

More than half of the parents (12) find the developments "concerning" or speak of a "dangerous" development. Five parents have a positive appreciation for the enhanced medical possibilities. They do however point out that all the available

Joop Stolk, Theo A. Boer & Ruth Seldenrijk (eds.). Meaningful Care, 127—139

choices make it more difficult for parents. Two parents do not state their opinions globally, but focus directly on selective abortions.

"Dangerous development"

Ann's parents call to mind a frightening image of parents who do not want their child, because it is inconvenient and too big a burden. Her mother expects that there will be much fewer children with a handicap in the future. That development reflects an increasing doubt about the meaning of these children's lives. She envisions a downward slope that reminds her of the Second World War. "Sometimes I say, 'this is like what happened with Hitler. He also wanted a perfect, unblemished people.' That just isn't possible in this broken world. It simply doesn't exist. I'm afraid that when we have conquered this, there will be something else. If one illness has been cured, another one will eventually pop up. Will we have to rise to different levels? Will mental retardation be the lowest level? Will people have to get smarter and smarter? It makes me shiver . . ."

John's mother finds it a frightening development, stating, "where do we draw the line?" His father is afraid of the slippery slope, "from my youth on, I have heard stories about the Second World War. Little by little, it became part of the law to have only the highest-functioning people remain. People were simply indoctrinated to decently remove the handicapped from society."

Tom's parents do not find the development in medical sciences bad "in and of itself". Their child has benefited from enhanced possibilities in medicine. But there are dangerous sides to this development. His mother states, "what I find dangerous is parents saying, 'this child is not wanted because of his handicap, let's have it removed.' You push away your own child, because something is wrong with him. It makes people more nonchalant, if it doesn't fit into their picture."

"Positive development with difficult choices"

Having the opportunity to have a prenatal exam is considered valuable by William's parents. "Yet," they say, "it doesn't make it any easier for parents." His father states, "there used to be a natural selection. William certainly wouldn't have made it back then. He would have died of blood poisoning within two days. You can be sure of that. Everyone would have said, 'well, it is for the best. Nature has decided. He probably wouldn't have amounted to anything, so it's better this way.'" Now, parents have to continually weigh the options and make difficult choices.

Jeffrey's mother also sees the benefits of medical developments. At the same time, she puts the possibilities into perspective: "I think the developments are good, but I know they really can't know everything. Just look at my situation; they weren't able to predict this . . ." His father thinks it is good that parents don't know everything: "we have talked about this and are glad we didn't know about it beforehand, because this way we didn't need to make that decision."

"Positive development"

Jim's mother stresses the positive developments. She sometimes thinks to herself, "I wish it were possible back then," to talk more openly about whether it would have been better to stop the medical care that Jim was receiving. "We have always said, 'it shouldn't have happened that way. Jim should have calmly passed away . . .' But I guess it has allowed us to really care for him during the past five years . . ."

Gertrud's mother thinks that the developments are "excellent". She especially appreciates the greater openness. "People have gotten more open and ask more questions. You can see it happening in the institution . . . there is much more talk about the possibilities . . ."

3. SELECTIVE ABORTION

With reference to their reaction to the opening question, we asked parents more closely about the prevention of handicaps by means of abortion. What do parents think about the possibility of prenatal testing and selective abortion? Would they, if needed, have a prenatal exam done? Would they, if given the choice, consider having an abortion? Were they ever given this option, and how did they choose?

Just a little over half of the parents (10 sets of parents, one father, and one mother) would not consider an abortion. Of these parents, four couples would make use of prenatal testing. The others did not consider a prenatal exam to be an acceptable or valuable option. Five sets of parents, one father, and one mother, would, after a prenatal exam and under specific conditions, choose to have an abortion. Two sets of parents had a prenatal exam with the goal of having an abortion if needed. One set of parents did indeed choose to have an abortion after finding out the results of the prenatal exam.

"No abortion, no prenatal testing"

Even if they were expecting a child with a handicap, John's parents would not consider terminating the pregnancy. His mother states, "I wouldn't dream of letting it be taken. Why not? I'm not sure why, but I could never do it. John is quite handicapped, but I wouldn't want to miss him for the world." His father adds, "Life is the most important thing there is. To take that away . . . The child might have had some joys in life, and we cut it off. I say this without a religious conviction; just as a human being. I think some people experience in one minute what others might not see their entire life . . . The value of life is unmeasurable."

Peter's mother doesn't find prenatal testing useful, "because we wouldn't do anything with it. We want to give the child a chance to be born. During the pregnancy, we already told each other, 'even if there is something wrong with the child, he is welcome.' It is our child, and we would like him to have the chance to be born." His father adds, "It might be easy to say that, but the moment you're faced with such a situation, it is very difficult indeed."

Stephen's parents faced a difficult choice in this matter. The metabolic disorder Stephen has, only affects boys, while girls simply would be carriers. His father says, "the dilemma was whether to have no more children after Stephen was born, or have children and accept them as they are, since we would never consider the third option: abortion. In our case, that would have meant aborting the boys, and keeping the girls . . . To abort the boys reminded us too much about the Jewish boys in

Egypt . . . It was either relinquish the dream of having more children, or take the risk and live with the consequences. We ended up choosing the second option." His parents had two more boys, without handicaps.

"Prenatal testing, but no abortion"

The parents of Hans oppose the idea of selective abortion. His mother says, "having a world with only perfect people is a bit too much . . ." She wouldn't mind someone having a prenatal exam to uncover potential defects, "if it puts the mother's mind at ease."

Gary's parents are also closed to the option of aborting a child. His mother states, "Are you only supposed to get good things in life? It isn't without purpose that you get something imperfect. That's how we see it, we should accept it. Should we only be happy if everyone is perfect?" His mother didn't feel well during her pregnancy with Gary. If it had been possible to have a prenatal exam, she would have had one done, "but we still would have had him."

"Abortion under certain circumstances"

Nearly a third of the parents isn't closed to the option of having a selective abortion. It is acceptable to end a pregnancy, depending on the gravity of the handicap. They have never faced this choice themselves, however.

For William's parents, the choice to have an abortion after a prenatal exam, depends on the nature of the handicap and on the expected quality of life. Testing for Down's Syndrome would, for that reason, not be an option for his mother. She states, "In that case, I would have the child." His father points out that there are situations which are much more dilemmatic, especially when much suffering for the child is involved: "When you see how a child degenerates, sometimes really fast, it suffers so badly . . ."

If the mother of Gertrud were to get pregnant again, and the fetus were diagnosed to have the same defect, she would choose to have an abortion. She wouldn't make this choice if the child were visually handicapped or blind. For her, the important consideration is whether the child will be able to live independently. The likelihood that a child with Down's Syndrome will not be able to live independently, would be reason for her to terminate the pregnancy.

Gertrud's father would want to distinguish between a high- and low-functioning child with Down's Syndrome. When asked about a possible discrepancy in his words, "I'm here for Gertrud." Regarding his wish to "prevent a child like Gertrud to be born," her father explains that with having just *one* child with a handicap, he is already drained of energy. "You're not able to care for more children with a handicap." Her mother adds, "what do you do with your own life? What are you doing to yourself? You certainly aren't on this earth to work yourself silly . . ."

If Paul's mother had known during the pregnancy that her child was going to be handicapped, she would have aborted it. "But," she adds, "he would have been an 'it' . . . not Paul, I didn't know him yet."

Choosing for abortion
Three of the mothers had a prenatal test done, because the parents were afraid that their next child would also be handicapped. In two instances, there was no handicap. One of the mothers, however, had a positive test result. The child would have the same serious metabolic disorder. The parents decided to end the pregnancy. The mother states, "we had very clearly agreed that if it had the same disorder, we would have it aborted. The results were positive. We couldn't believe our ears. You basically start with the assumption that everything will be okay. It was terrible . . . But I really am glad I saved it the suffering that I see my son go through. I have never regretted making that choice . . ."

4. LIMITS IN THE MEDICAL CARE OF CHILDREN WITH PROFOUND MULTIPLE HANDICAPS

4.1. Introduction

"Children with profound multiple handicaps are vulnerable. They are often ill. Should everything be done, in the case of serious illness, to save this child's life, or should there be limits to medical intervenion. If so, what are these limits? Have you ever found yourself in those limits with the care of your child? Does the institution where your child resides have any policies regarding starting or ceasing treatment?"

Parents didn't have a simple answer to these questions. After all, it concerns complex subject matter and deep-reaching events in the lives of the parents. Often, these questions led to "thinking out loud", and carefully coming to a conclusion. Several parents answered the questions with a question, without coming to a direct answer. When trying to identify possible limits, some parents noted that "when reality strikes, everything can suddenly look different."

The answers given by the parents cannot be placed into simple categories, such as "for-or-against life termination". There were too many nuances in their answers for that. We will share the words of ten (randomly picked) parents regarding possible limits in medical care. Then we will give an overview of their reactions to the question whether their child's institution has any policies regarding limits in medical care.

4.2. Limits in Medical Care?

"William"
William was quite ill shortly after birth, and his parents had their doubts whether his care should be continued. His mother remembers, "you see this little hump of a person lying there and wonder, 'how will things turn out? Maybe it would be better to . . .'" His father finishes, ". . . perhaps it would be better to stop giving him blood and to let it all end." Now, years later, his parents are able to say that they had these thoughts because they had not bonded with their child yet. His mother recalls that "all that time, we didn't have a chance to hold him." His father has the same memory: "It all seemed so far removed . . ." The parents are glad that at that time, and later, they never had to make the choice to stop a medical treatment. "Imagine,"

his father states, "that at a given point you say, 'I think it has been enough now,' and that the doctor responds, 'well, if you think so . . .'" William's mother adds, ". . . that would stay with you your whole life: what would have become of him?" His father responds, "exactly; at least we can say that we did all we could . . ."

"Patrick"
Patrick's father would definitely not want to keep a newborn with profound multiple handicaps alive at all costs. "If you have a child with serious defects, and don't really have a strong bond with it yet, you really shouldn't go to all lengths to keep it alive. That wouldn't be wise. I sometimes wonder whether Medicine hasn't progressed too far in a number of areas. These children would never have survived a hundred years ago. Newer and better medical treatments just keep piling up . . . Whereas life often could not be sustained in the past, now it has become possible in many situations, thanks to the medical sciences. That is the hard part: where are the limits?" Evenso, if at that time his father had known what he knows now, he would not have acted differently, because Patrick was not sick as a newborn. "It would have been different if he had had spina bifida. In that case, I would probably have reacted otherwise. But he was really a normal baby, just a little small."

"Jim"
Jim's parents talk about their son's long history of illnesses. His mother explains how "he has suffered enormously. The doctors have warned us that if Jim becomes that ill again, he will continuously need to receive oxygen and won't be able to eat anymore." If it reaches that point, his mother believes they have reached a limit: "at one point you have to draw the line between a worthy human life and a greenhouse plant. My feelings tell me that I don't want to lose him. But my mind tells me differently. And in such a situation, you should act on what your mind tells you." Jim's father says, "at that point you know how long it will last. But attaching him to a continuous oxygen flow like a greenhouse plant . . . We told ourselves, 'he has already struggled so hard in the five years of his life, that continuing this battle simply because we cannot stand being without him, no, it just wouldn't be right . . .'" His mother remembers how "they kept him alive when he was born. They should have never done that. I often stood at his bedside, thinking, 'maybe I should pull out all this mess, all these tubes and machines. But they never gave us that choice . . .' We have always said, 'it shouldn't have happened this way; Jim should have gently fallen asleep . . .' But, oh well, on the other hand . . . these past five years we have, in some ways, really been able to enjoy him."

"Tom"
Tom's parents cannot imagine that they would ever say to a doctor, "in this or that circumstance, stop treating him." That would be contradictory to what they once promised their son, namely, to "always fight for him." This has made for quite a battle, about which his mother says the following: "on the one hand, we have prayed that he would no longer be here. But when push came to shove, our actions spoke differently: when Tom became ill, we were nearly fanatical in fighting for his life. I

remember thinking, 'how does this figure?' We decided that if the Lord decides to take him, it is good. But I don't want him to die by our own doing . . . When Tom's health worsens, we both analyze why it is getting worse, and what we can do about it. This has happened many times, and each time we found that there was a reason for it. One time he had terrible medication toxicity. As parents, we knew that something was wrong. We told ourselves, 'he needs to go to the hospital.'" His father adds, "we made our demands clear to the physician: 'this is what needs to be done, and if you don't do it, there will be trouble.'" His mother continues, "in a situation like that, you don't want to lose him . . . If the Lord were to say, 'Tom, okay, it's time to come home,' it would be fine, no problem . . . But until now, we have only faced situations where Tom was threatening to die because of human errors. Under such conditions, all that is in us wants to fight for his life."

"Beth"
Beth's mother thinks about the other children in Beth's group who have died: "I don't know if I would have fought so long to extend their lives. I can say that now, but of course I'm not facing the choice myself." Her father remembers the times when Beth was seriously ill: "a moment might come where we'll have to say, 'it won't work.' When children with profound handicaps truly suffer, it might be up to the parent to say, 'let's talk to the physician and discuss if we really should keep treating this.'" For Beth's mother, "pain really is the limit. I don't want her to have a tremendous amount of pain. I have always thought about the possibility of letting her die, but when Beth was very ill, I thought for the first time that it might be best for the doctors to actively intervene . . ." Her father continues, "at the same time you realize that it would be very drastic to intervene in that way . . ." He believes that once a child is born, it should be cared for. His stand is: "abortion, yes; euthanasia, in principle no, unless the child is to die within a short amount of time anyway." Beth's father isn't sure whether he could ever choose for euthanasia: "be very careful in making a decision to end someone's life; you can see how happy Beth is . . . Such a decision should never be made because the handicapped child doesn't fit into your pretty picture of the world. That is not a valid reason. The choice should be based on the child's life expectancy and the problems it might have when kept alive."

"Mark"
Mark had an accident while playing. He was admitted to the hospital with serious oxygen deprivation. His condition was critical. His father remembers, "they even told us, 'we will resuscitate him only one more time. If that does not work, it is over . . ." Mark's mother finds it "a wonder that we still have him with us." At the hospital, his parents were at times criticized for what they wanted to be done for Mark. "They would say, 'do you know what you are getting in to?'" His mother states, "giving him nothing to eat was something we couldn't bring ourselves to." "At one point," says his father, "we said, 'if he can only be kept alive by artificial means, then he has the right to die.' He was removed from the respirator. The doctor asked us, 'if he doesn't make it, what do you want us to do? Put him back on the

respirator? Or does he also have the right to die?' We decided to let him die if he didn't breathe on his own . . . If God calls him home, who are we to say, 'come on, he should stay hooked to that machine.'"

"Gary"

Gary's mother doubts whether it is possible to give a clear prognosis at the time a child with a handicap is born: "who could make that prediction? With our Gary, they told us, 'don't make any assumptions.' I don't think that the physician knew what would become of him either. And now look how he has developed, even beyond our own expectations." His father believes that "you should try everything to keep the child alive. If it dies in a normal fashion, then I would have peace with it, but don't perform euthanasia . . ." His mother adds, "if Gary were to become very ill, the same should be done for him as for any other child, any normal child . . ."

"Helen"

According to Helen's parents, it was "by force" that she was kept alive by her physicians after her birth. When Helen was ill again recently, she fought to stay alive. Her mother says, "this time she wanted it herself. I had wanted to act in order to allow her to die. She had a very serious intestinal infection. She refused any food for three days. She refused every drop or bite. She was gravely ill. She had a fever of 107°F. But after many difficult discussions, we decided, 'no, we will offer her something now and then. If she wants to, she can stay alive.' And indeed, after a number of really tough days, it seemed she was coming back. A week later, she fell into a deep sleep. She slept continuously for three nights and days. We thought that this was probably the coma phase; 'if she leaves us now, we will let her go. We will not force it.' During those days, we had some tough discussions with each other about the best approach. Should she go to the hospital? You could say that she made her own choice this time. It was the first time we experienced this. She chose to keep going . . . I think I would have gone a step further. I wouldn't have offered her any more food. I would have let her slip away, dehydrate, and let her go . . . We knew she would be placed in an institution soon. To me, that was even more awful than dying . . . worse than just letting her slip away. She had already lost a lot of weight and was dehydrated; she was already far gone . . . Imagine that she would go into another deep sleep like that, I think I could do it this time: offer her no more fluids, medicate her so that she'll keep sleeping, until she is able to move on . . . Of course, the aftermath would be more difficult for me, but I'd rather have a hard time than watch her suffer an unliveable life." The parents are of one mind in this regard. Helen's father states, "my wife has more courage than I do. I was more prone to offer her fluids. I'm not sure whether it was love, or cowardice. Let me put it this way: if she had passed away, I would be at peace with it . . ."

"Ann"

Ann's father is afraid that the developments in Medicine will lead to endless lengthening of life. "I wonder if that is God's purpose. He gives people knowledge in order to do a thing or two. That is good, but if that were to continue without limit

. . ." Her father and mother try to identify their limits while talking. Does the limit lie at tube feeding? At ventilation? In the end, they create their own formula: one should not actively terminate a life, but must be very careful not to extend a life at all costs. Later during the conversation, Ann's father finds a mid-way point. Whether one must never terminate a life, is not so clear to him. He doesn't exclude the possibility. He states, "I could imagine that there are exceptions, but it should only be allowed in extraordinary situations." At the same time, he points out that there are "bad people" who do not want their child, because it is a nuisance to them. "That, to me, is terrifying."

"Larry"

A number of weeks before the interview with his parents took place, Larry died. His mother recalls how difficult it had always been to make all the decisions for him and to never be able to ask him what he wanted himself. She states, "the last few weeks, we were faced with the question of what to do if Larry were to suffocate, whether we should resuscitate him at that point. I am glad and thankful that I never had to make the decision to put him on a respirator; what if he couldn't come off of it, and we would have to pull the plug? That would have been incredibly difficult for me. I'm glad we were saved from making that decision." Larry's mother tells us about a doctor with whom she had a conflict several years ago. Larry had pneumonia, and a collapsed lung. "The doctor said, 'we ought to call it a day.' I got very mad, because I knew that downstairs, in the department with all the incubators, there were little one-pound babies, as small as barbie dolls. I saw how they were being kept alive, at all costs . . . But they don't know what the future of a one-pound baby holds, and how its little brain will develop. At one point, I put this doctor in a difficult spot: 'you want to call it a day for Larry . . . We don't know what the future will bring, but I think he has exactly the same rights as a little one-pound baby, for whom you also don't know what the future will hold.' He told me, 'you use harsh words.' I said, 'yes, perhaps I have to. You want to call it a day, I don't . . . I want to have an answer *now*.' He said, 'that, I can't give you.' I insisted, 'I want to have an answer *now*. Will you help my boy or not? You do help other newborns downstairs!' He got very quiet and white as a ghost and said, 'does he mean that much to you?' 'yes,' I said, 'he is everything to us.' He said, 'then I will do all I can.' Larry then received a gastrostomy. He lived with it for six more years. He gained 50 pounds. Yes, I was very harsh with that doctor. I even said, 'if you have a child like this in your care, don't just look at what you see lying in front of you, but also look at what the child means to the parents. Think about it, before you make such a quick judgment.' The doctor told us he had learned a lot from us."

4.3. Agreements with the Institution

Along with the questions regarding the limits of medical care, parents were asked whether any agreements had been made with their son's or daughter's institution regarding the starting or ending of a medical treatment.

Nineteen children have been placed out of the home. For six of these children, there is an agreement with the institution. Parents and physicians have met, and jointly determined where the limits are in regard to deciding whether to treat or not (or to stop treatment). One set of parents doesn't think it necessary to make such an arrangement, because they "fully trust" the institution. One set of parents does not want to make an arrangement, because it would feel like they are betraying their son. The remaining parents have not made an agreement because there either is no urgency, or because they find the subject too difficult.

For three of the parents who have made arrangements, the limit is at "artificial respiration". David's parents have agreed with the physicians that he will never receive respirator assistance. They thought about it for a long time. They made this difficult decision after consulting with their daughter, who is a nurse. David also wouldn't be able to handle it because of his handicap. Physically, he has too much spasticity, and mentally he couldn't handle it either. His mother says, "we're afraid that once he is started on a respirator, he will never be able to get off. We hope that it will all go naturally' . . . Of course we want to do all we can. To give him the needed care. We won't say, 'well, it has been enough.' No, we want to do all that is necessary." His father adds, "we pray that the Lord will guide things in such a way, that the question won't have to be asked, that we won't have to make that decision."

For two parents, the limit lies at "resuscitation", and they have indicated this to the institution. Art's parents believe that their son's life does not need to be artificially extended. According to his father, "there have been a few occasions in which he stopped breathing. Twice, he really needed help. But we have said that we don't want him admitted to a hospital anymore, and that they don't need to go to all ends to save his life. They should allow him to die peacefully. Don't end up doing some heart massage, and another heart massage, so that he'll end up with broken ribs, bleeding in his lungs, and all sorts of other complications. If he is to die, then let him die in peace. Let us look at it soberly. If he stops, his time has come."

One set of parents has set the limit at the administration of antibiotics. After their son had one pneumonia after the other, with serious complications, they don't see the need to "go to all means to prevent his death again."

5. INFLUENCES ON THE PARENTS' THINKING

Never before have the media put the issue of moral dilemmas in the health care of children with profound multiple handicaps in the limelight like they do today. The issue is brought up in every possible news medium, including the Internet. The parents were asked whether this public debate, in particular when it pertains to the prevention of handicaps, has influenced their personal views, and whether it has affected the way in which they accept their child.

5.1. Influence on Personal Views

Two parents were not asked this particular question. Two parents stated that they do not follow this public discussion, because "it doesn't get you anywhere". Five parents stated that articles or programs on this subject do not influence them. They do read and listen to them, but their viewpoint has not changed.

Brian's mother states that she does hear and watch these programs, but that they don't cause her to think about her own child. The story of her own child, she feels, simply is different, and therefore she cannot relate. "Those people don't know what they're talking about. I'd like to have them spend a week in an institution so they can learn what joy these people experience in their lives."

Peter's parents follow the discussions with great interest. His mother notes, "before, when I used to hear such programs, I only listened with half an ear. But now, when the subject, 'handicapped', is mentioned, we immediately turn up the radio or television." The programs make these parents think. "We were just talking about limits. I think this will always be difficult. Sometimes I think, 'if he had been born fifty years ago, he wouldn't be alive anymore.' That can be pretty tough . . . In that regard, it used to be easier." When asked whether the programs brought her into confusion, she answered, "if someone is down in the dumps and hears and reads all those things, I could imagine that at some point they wouldn't know what to think anymore, or maybe even what to feel anymore . . . When we hear the parents on those programs say, 'it would be better if it came to an end,' we can really relate to how they are feeling."

Four parents note how the discussion about the limits of medical care has "alerted" them to possible abuse of those limits. Ann's mother states, "I'm all over them, when Ann is in the hospital. I want to know all their plans."

The publicity around the (medical) care of children with profound multiple handicaps doesn't leave the parents unaffected. Four parents state that the discussions hurt them. Three parents say that they can get very angry, and two parents say that they have great difficulty with the "mentality behind the discussion."

Art's mother can get angry about the discussion around abortion. This discussion is to her a proclamation that children born with a handicap do not have the right to live. What also causes her anger is that it does not only concern the handicap, but that it is also a financial issue: ". . . it all comes down to money."

Taylor's parents see the difficulty people have with a child with a handicap as a consequence of the "spirit of this age". His mother says, "I tend to think that in this day and age, people have such small hearts. They don't want to give up a thing, everything revolves around the self: 'as long as things go well for us, as long as we . . .' We can't seem to make sacrifices anymore. At least, that is my impression. It isn't only this way with these children, but also with caring for anyone. We sacrifice everything for our car, our house . . ." His father adds, "it's true; just as my wife said, we seem to live in a very egocentric world. People have no concern for their fellow man. I think it is related to our wealth, our culture. That strikes me about this world: people aren't willing to help each other anymore . . . The question is whether we still want to pay the price for a handicapped child, whether we want to give it a chance to live, or whether we say, 'no, he doesn't fit in this world. Take it away.'"

5.2. Influence on the Acceptance of the Child

Does the discussion about selective abortion and selective (non-)treatment of newborn children with profound multiple handicaps make it more difficult for parents to accept their own child? Behind this question lies the thought that with the new possibilities in preventing handicaps, parents might be led to doubt the meaning of their child's life, and the meaning of caring for their child. If it isn't a matter of course anymore to let children with handicaps be born, parents could come to think that all the labour and care they have given to their child would not have been necessary if they had (could have) made a different choice back then.

Two parents were not asked this question. More than half of the remaining parents (11) state that this discussion has not influenced their acceptance of their child. These parents state that they have accepted their child, and that outsiders cannot change that. Most of these parents give a direct answer, stating "no", "absolutely not", or, "I couldn't imagine". A few parents don't provide an answer.

If the public discussion really has such an influence, Brian's mother would consider that "stupid, very stupid." "That would be sad, because it would mean that some people listen more to other voices than to their own. I love my child, and no one could possibly change that. Brian simply belongs to the family, that's how it has always been."

Helen's parents are encouraged by the fact that this discussion is taking place. Her mother states, "we have fought for Helen in a time when Medicine ruled, when these sorts of questions were rarely asked." The parents themselves are repeatedly confronted with questions about the limits of Medicine. They have put much thought into where these limits lie. Whether or not to accept their child was not an issue, however. Her mother states, "I consider that a different subject . . ."

According to seven parents, the debate in the newspapers, on the radio, and on television, makes it more difficult for parents to accept their child. Two of these parents speak from experience. The remaining parents recall what they have heard other parents say.

Mark's parents could imagine that some parents might have difficulty accepting their child. They themselves have experienced much sadness in this regard, but as parents, they couldn't let it discourage them. His father says, "well, I can imagine it. But we just tell ourselves, 'what good does it do? You can doubt, you can worry, but you can't change the way things are.' We have to deal with it, this is simply the road we must take. We have to make the best of it. That's how we see it."

David's parents believe it has become increasingly difficult to accept a child with a handicap, especially for young parents. His mother says, "when David was born, that simply wasn't an issue yet. I think it is difficult for many young parents when they know before the birth that their child will be handicapped. They have a choice to make. What incredible tension that must create!"

Two parents state that they themselves haven't been influenced by the discussion, but that they do notice that people with a handicap are less and less accepted in society. Ann's mother recalls how once she was waiting in line at the grocery store, with her daughter in the wheelchair. Behind her stood a pregnant woman. "I thought, 'she would probably like to put her stuff down.' So I told her, 'wait, I'll move over.' She didn't say a word; she simply ignored me. Then I heard the mother standing next to her say, 'that they allow a child like that to be born.' My heart sunk. I was at a loss for words. I just went home. When I got home, I told myself, 'I will never take her out again . . .'"

6. CONCLUDING REMARKS

There is an intricate interaction between developments and opinions in society as a whole, and the decisions and experiences of parents. This interaction cannot be described in simple terms. If our qualitative survey indicates something, it is how different the reactions of parents can be. Some seem to be strongly opposed to any suggestions that the birth or life of a child with a handicap should be prevented by medical means, such as genetic screening, prenatal diagnosis, non-treatment decisions, or euthanasia. Others, however, are more prone to accept at least some of these options as a way to prevent handicaps and suffering. In general, however, it seems clear that parents of a child with mental retardation are somewhat more critical towards medical techniques to prevent the birth of a child with a handicap, than are those who do not speak from personal experience. For many parents, experiences of meaning in caring for their child are the basis for this conviction (*Cf.* chapter two of this book).

Of course, the interaction between society and parents, as the word suggests, goes both ways: not only are parents of children with mental retardation influenced by developments and opinions in society, but there is also an opposite movement: parents — and potential parents — influence the way in which society as a whole reflects upon the prevention of handicaps. To what extent this is true, will have to be the object of a future survey.

SECTION FOUR

EXPERIENCE OF MEANING IN DAILY CARE

STANLEY M. HAUERWAS

CHAPTER 10

TIMEFUL FRIENDS

Living with People with Mental Retardation[*]

1. INTRODUCTION: L'ARCHE

"L'Arche is special, in the sense that we are trying to live in community with people who are mentally handicapped. Certainly we want to help them grow and reach the greatest independence possible. But before 'doing for them', we want to 'be with them'. The particular suffering of the person who is mentally handicapped, as of all marginal people, is a feeling of being excluded, worthless and unloved. It is through everyday life in community and the love that must be incarnate in this, that handicapped people can begin to discover that they have a value, that they are loved and so are lovable."[1]

"Individual growth towards love and wisdom is slow. A community's growth is even slower. Members of a community have to be friends of time. They have to learn that many things will resolve themselves if they are given enough time. It can be a great mistake to want, in the name of clarity and truth, to push things too quickly to a resolution. Some people enjoy confrontation and highlighting divisions. This is not always healthy. It is better to be a friend of time. But clearly too, people should not pretend that problems don't exist by refusing to listen to the rumblings of discontent; they must be aware of the tensions."[2]

"Our focal point of fidelity at l'Arche is to live with handicapped people in the spirit of the Gospel and the Beatitudes. 'To live with' is different from 'to do for'. It doesn't simply mean eating at the same table and sleeping under the same roof. It means that we create relationships of gratuity, truth and interdependence, that we listen to the handicapped people, that we recognize and marvel at their gifts. The day we become no more than professional workers and educational therapists is the day we stop being l'Arche — although of course 'living with' does not exclude this professional aspect."[3]

2. ON THE ETHICS OF WRITING ABOUT THE ETHICS OF THE CARE OF PEOPLE WITH MENTAL RETARDATION

Every time I write about people with mental retardation I make a promise to myself that it will be the last time I write about this subject. Yet here I am breaking my promise once again. I published my first essay on people with mental retardation

[*] First published in: Stanley Hauerwas, *Sanctify Them in the Truth*. Edinburgh: T&T Clark, 1998. Reprinted with permission.

Joop Stolk, Theo A. Boer & Ruth Seldenrijk (eds.). Meaningful Care, 143—154

over twenty years ago. I have continued to speak and write about them ever since. Surely, one would think, by now I have said all I have to say. Of course, such an attitude, that is, that I have said what I have to say, is that of an intellectual. Those who really care about people with mental retardation never run out of things to say, since they do not write "about" people with mental retardation precisely because they do not view them as just another "subject". They write for and in some sense with people with mental retardation.

To be able to write for and with people with mental retardation requires that you know people who are mentally handicapped. By "know" I mean you must be *with* them in a way they may be able to claim you as a friend. I was once so claimed, but over the last few years I have not enjoyed such a friendship. So when I now write about the ethics of caring for people with mental retardation, I fear I am not talking about actual people but more of my memories of people with mental retardation. When they become an abstraction, moreover, we can begin to think we must provide "reasons" for their existence or, worse, discover meaning in why we care for them. As the passages I quoted at the beginning make clear, Jean Vanier feels no need to find meaning in why l'Arche homes exist.

I call attention to the tension I feel in yet once again writing about people with mental retardation, because my difficulty illustrates the challenge facing all who care for them. How do we care for people with mental retardation without allowing the reasons we are tempted to give for such care to distort what should be our relation to those for whom we care? To make the question even more difficult — "How do we care for people with mental retardation in such a manner which would forestall our felt need to provide reasons why we should care for people with mental retardation, thereby rendering their lives unintelligible?" After all, both the existence and care of those of us who are considered "normal" is not thought to require justification. Why is the existence and/or care of the "mentally handicapped" singled out as presenting a special problem?

In truth my difficulty about writing about people with mental retardation did not begin with my isolation from them. From the beginning I have always felt a bit duplicitous when I addressed the subject of the mentally handicapped and their care. In fact, I have not ever really written about people with mental retardation. No matter how much I care for them, I have been haunted by the presumption that my "interest" in them and my writing about them has been part of an intellectual agenda that makes them useful to me. Once I had been drawn into the world of people with mental retardation, however, it did not take me long to realize they were the crack I desperately needed to give concreteness to my critique of modernity. No group exposes the pretensions of the humanism that shapes the practices of modernity more thoroughly than people with mental retardation.

Our humanism entails we care for them once they are among us, once we are stuck with them; but the same humanism cannot help but think that, all things considered, it would be better if they did not exist. As modern people we think we are meant to be autonomous beings. In view of such an overpowering presumption, how do we make sense of those among us whose very existence can be nothing but dependence? We live in cultures for which rationality and consciousness are taken to be the very essence of what makes us human. What are we to make of those who will never, even with the best efforts, be able to read or write? Should they be considered human?

Examples of how people with mental retardation render problematic some of the most cherished conceits of modernity are legion. For example, in his *Life As We Know It: A Father, a Family, and an Exceptional Child*, Michael Berube tells of the birth and care he and his wife have given to their son Jamie, who has Down's Syndrome. His is a wonderful story of how two college professors found their lives reshaped by their son's disability. I have nothing but admiration for the way they have accepted and cared for their son. The story Berube tells of their struggle to keep Jamie alive and to secure appropriate medical care is at once as inspiring as it is humane.

Moreover, professor Berube has read his Foucault. He knows that some of the most humane forms of "treatment" may be but forms of control. He even knows that the most humane accounts of justice in modernity, such as those of Rawls and Habermas, cannot help his son. That such accounts of justice require that we shed our individual idiosyncrasies make the existence of his son irresolvably problematic. As Berube puts it,

> There isn't a chance in the world that James Lyon Berube could come to the table independently of "interests", independent of cognitive and social idiosyncrasies legible to all, independent of either a genetic makeup or a social apparatus that constructs him as "abnormal". The society that fosters Jamie's independence must start from an understanding of his dependencies, and any viable conception of justice has to take the concrete bodies and "private", idiosyncratic interest of individuals like Jamie into account, or it will be of no account at all.[4]

Berube criticizes Rawls and Habermas for succumbing to "a curious Enlightenment fantasy, the idea that once we boil away all the idiosyncrasies and impurities of the irrational human race, we can come up with some perfectly neutral, rational, disinterested character who can play the language-game of justice as if it were a contest in which he or she had no stake."[5] Yet Berube's criticism of Rawls and Habermas rings hollow in the light of his own narrative. He either cannot or does not choose to make intelligible his admirable commitment to Jamie.

For example, with great candor Berube tells us that he and his wife are as pro-choice after the birth of Jamie as they were prior to his birth. Indeed, he notes that they intentionally did not use amniocentesis, assuming they would "just love the baby all the more" if the baby was born with Down's Syndrome. He confesses such a stance was "blithe and uninformed" and that if they had known that their child's life "would be suffering and misery for all concerned" they might have chosen to have an abortion."[6] Berube notes, however, that it is extremely difficult to discuss Jamie in this way. Just as it was hard to talk about him as a medicalized being when he was in the ICU, it is still harder "to talk about him in terms of our philosophical beliefs about abortion and prenatal testing. That's partly because these issues are so famously divisive and emotionally charged, but it's also because we can no longer frame any such questions about our child now that he's here."[7]

"Now that he is here" is the nub of the matter. Berube does not pretend to be able to do more than represent Jamie "now that he is here". Indeed, he takes that as his ethical and aesthetic task — to help us imagine Jamie and to imagine what he might think of our ability to imagine him. Just as the Berubes look forward to the day that Jamie will be able to eat at the "big" table, to feed himself tacos, burgers, and pizza, to set the table even if such a setting is somewhat "random", so Berube's job "is to represent my son, to set his place at our collective table. But I know I am merely trying my best to prepare for the day he sets his own place. For I have no sweeter dream than to imagine — aesthetically and ethically and parentally — that Jamie will someday be his own advocate, his own author, his own best representative."[8]

How sad. All Berube can imagine for Jamie is that he be "his own author". That Berube can imagine no other future is not his fault. His imagination but reflects the same limits that formed the conceptions of justice he found so unsatisfactory. What other possibility could there be in a world in which God does not exist? What other politics is available for those like the Berubes when the church has been reduced to reinforcing the sentimentalities of contemporary humanism? Berube has been gifted with Jamie, but he lacks the practices of a community that would provide the resources for narrating his own and Jamie's life.

That is the "crack" I have exploited in the interest of a theological agenda. In short, I have used the "now that he is here" as a resource to illumine Christian speech. Christians know that we have not been created to be "our own authors", to be autonomous. We are creatures. Dependency, not autonomy, is one of the ontological characteristics of our lives. That we are creatures, moreover, is but a reminder that we are created for and with one another. We are not just accidentally communal, but we are such by necessity. We were not created to be alone. We cannot help but desire and delight in the reality of the other, even the other born with a difference we call mental retardation.

Our dependency, our need for one another, means that we will suffer as well as know joy. Our incompleteness at once makes possible the gifts that make life possible as well as the unavoidability of suffering. Such suffering, moreover, may seem pointless. Yet, at least for Christians, such suffering should not tempt us to think our task is to eliminate those whose suffering seems pointless.[9] Christians are, or at least should be, imbedded in a narrative that makes possible a sharing of our lives with one another that enables us to go on in the face of the inexplicable.

For Christians people with mental retardation do not present a peculiar challenge. That people with mental retardation are constituted by narratives they have not chosen but reveals the character of our lives. That some people are born with a condition that we have come to label as being mentally retarded does not indicate a fundamental difference between them and the fact that we must all be born. The question is not whether we can justify people with mental retardation, but whether we live any longer in a world that can make sense of having children. At the very least, Christians believe that our lives are constituted by the hope we have learned through Christ's cross and resurrection that makes morally intelligible the bringing children into a world as dark as our own.

I have not made these arguments to try to convince people constituted by the narratives of modernity that they should believe in God. Such an argument could not help but make God a *deus ex machina* which not only demeans God, but God's creation as well. Rather, my concern is to help Christians locate those practices that help us understand better why our willingness to welcome people with mental retardation should not be surprising given the triune nature of the God we worship. In other words, I have used people with mental retardation as material markers necessary to show that Christian speech can and in fact does make claims about the way things are. Theologically thinking about people with mental retardation helps us see, moreover, that claims about the way things are cannot be separated from the way we should live.

By subjecting people with mental retardation to this agenda, one might object, am I not also exemplifying the desperate attempt I have criticized in others to find some "meaning" in the existence and care of people with mental retardation? I would obviously like to answer with a quick denial, but as I indicated above, the question rightly continues to haunt me. That it does so, I think, is partly because I am not sure how one rightly responds to such a challenge. What sense are we to make of the care given to people with mental retardation in a world of limited resources? I think the answer requires the reshaping of the question — a reshaping, I believe, gestured at in the work of people like Jean Vanier. For we will only know why we do what we do by the exemplary lives of those like Vanier who teach us how to live with those we call people with mental retardation. So I can do no better than to turn our attention to his work.

3. ON "USING" PEOPLE WITH MENTAL RETARDATION

Before I turn to Vanier, however, I want to expose a narrative that I suspect may inform and shape questions about the "use" of people with mental retardation — that is, the kind of problematic that has shaped what I have just said about my own dis-ease with my use of people with mental retardation. It is, moreover, a narrative that I think is particularly pernicious, not only for the care of people with mental retardation, but for any human relations, including our relations to animals and nature. This narrative received its most eloquent expression as well as its most adequate defense in the second formulation of Kant's categorical imperative — "Act so that you treat humanity, whether in your own person or in that of another, always as an end and never as a means only."[10]

For many such an imperative seems to embody our highest ideal. Kant certainly did not think of it as an ideal, but rather thought such an imperative constitutive of any moral act that deserves the description, "moral". Unfortunately this results in the creation of the realm of "morality" that moderns assume can be distinguished from economics, politics, or, more importantly, manners. Once such a realm exists, some people then think they have to think about the "ethics" of the care of the retarded.

The power of this narrative, that is, that we should treat one another as ends and not means, is revealed for modern people by the very fact we cannot imagine anyone seriously challenging it as a statement of what we should at least always try to do. One may doubt the existence of God, but it seems everyone agrees that we ought never to treat one another simply as an end. The way we often put the matter is that every human being should be treated with dignity. Of course, like most abstractions, it is very hard to know what it means to treat others as ends. That most human relations require we treat one another as means does not seem to call into question the assumption that we ought not to do so. Whatever the difficulty may be in concrete specification of treating another as an end, we continue to think we all would prefer to be treated as an end not a means.

This seems particularly to be the case when it comes to people with mental retardation. We presume that the improvement in the care of people with mental retardation over this century derives from our commitment to treat them as persons deserving respect — that is, as ends in themselves. There is, of course, the troubling problem of whether people with mental retardation possess the characteristics necessary to be counted as persons. If they do not, for example, possess minimal forms of rationality, can they be considered persons deserving respect? Is the care of such beings then to be considered supererogatory? Such questions may be considered too theoretical to be of interest, but if resources become scarce, questions about the care of people with mental retardation can begin to have frightening implications.

The language of means and ends often has peculiar power in the treatment people with mental retardation actually receive. The ethic that often shapes critiques of institutionalization of people with mental retardation, that creates the demand for their normalization, that requires they receive appropriate medical treatment, is one that assumes they too should be treated as ends not as "means only".[11] That any restrictions on people with mental retardation should be the "least restrictive" seems to require that people with mental retardation are to be treated as far as possible like anyone else.

Yet what "as far as possible" means is not easily determined. For example, Michael Berube observes how the Foucauldian question haunts the humanities:

> Is it wrong to speak for others, to assume that one can represent the interests of another in a faithful and transparent way? How can one be an advocate for the mentally retarded while believing that institutions never die and that every act of representation is also an act of usurpation? Is there no way to have faith in Camelot, in Special Olympics, in Advocacy?[12]

Berube answers that whatever he may believe about the history of madness, sexuality, incarceration, it is impossible to act as a Foucauldian when it comes to Jamie.

> We have to act, for both theoretical and practical reasons, in the belief that these agencies can benefit our child, even as the sorry history of institutionalization weighs on our brains like a nightmare. To act in any other way, to indict all such institutions across the board, would be to consign Jamie to the kind of self-fulfilling prophecy that follows from unearned cynicism: We know they can't help, so why bother? It would be hard to imagine a more irresponsible attitude toward his life's prospects.[13]

Yet Berube knows, as every parent of people with mental retardation knows, that they are caught in what seems an irresolvable conundrum. In order for your child to receive appropriate care they must be labeled — retarded, handicapped, Down's Syndrome — but the labels can become self-fulfilling prophecies; or worse, the labels can legitimate the intervention of others into their children's lives that often only benefits the agents of intervention. This becomes particularly troubling when the agent of intervention is an institution called the state. Parents want their child treated as an end, with respect, but in a social ethos dominated by an ethic of respect their children can only be treated as a means.

Which I think brings us back to Kant and why the second formulation of the categorical imperative is not only inadequate to help us understand the place of people with mental retardation but for any account of morality. For what is often forgotten is that Kant's formulation of the categorical imperative presupposes an account of existence that is without ultimate *telos*. What purpose there is results from human freedom now understood as an end in itself. Humanity is forced to impose meaning on a mechanistic world whose only meaning is to be found in our existence as humans. Human behaviour is subject to mechanistic explanation as any part of nature. We remain ends only to the extent we can will ourselves to be such.

What such a view of the world cannot do is to allow us to ask, "What are people for?"[14] Such a question presupposes that creation, all that is, has a purpose that is not a function of our self-generating will. On such a view human beings have a *telos* that allows a distinction to be drawn between "man-as-he-happens-to-be and man-as-he-could-be-if-he-realized-his-essential-nature. Ethics is the science which is to enable men to understand how they make the transition from the former state to the latter."[15] Such a transition, moreover, requires a community, and the purpose of the community for which we are created is nothing less than friendship with one another.

From such a perspective we can begin to appreciate how few resources the means-ends manner of thinking provides for helping us understand the care of people with mental retardation. Of course, we "use" people with mental retardation, but we are here to be of use to one another. The notion that any use we make of one another can only be justified if it is done voluntarily can now be seen as one of the peculiar sentimentalities of modernity that results in self-supervision all the more tyrannical since what we do is allegedly what we want to do. That people with mental retardation are subject to care for their own good — a good they may not have chosen — is not an indication that such care is misguided, but rather requires that the goods that such care is serving be properly named. After all, they (like us who are not retarded) exist to serve and to be served for our mutual upbuilding.

As Christians we should not feel embarrassed to discover that people with mental retardation among us help us better understand the narrative that constitutes the very purpose of our existence. That such is the case does not "justify" their existence, but then their existence no more than our existence from a Christian perspective requires justification. We are free to help them just to the extent we no longer feel the necessity to justify their existence. The form such "help" takes can only be discovered relative to the tasks of the community necessary to sustain the practices for the discovery and care of the goods held in common. Put in terms I used above, Christians do not use people with mental retardation as an affront to a world without purpose, but we should not be surprised that the Christian refusal to abandon people with mental retardation to such a world will be seen as an affront.

We must confess as Christians, however, that our care of people with mental retardation has been shaped more by the means/end narrative than by that of Christ. As a result, in the name of care we too often subject people with a handicap to therapies based on mechanistic presumptions that promise "results" rather than community. That is why the alternative Vanier represents is so important. For l'Arche offers an imaginative portrayal of what a purposive community might look like in which people with mental retardation serve and are served.[16]

4. VANIER'S WISDOM

I am aware, of course, that I will be accused of romanticizing Vanier and the l'Arche movement. Yet as Vanier reminds us,

> Too many communities are founded on dreams and fine words; there is much talk about love, truth, and peace. Marginal people are demanding. Their cries are cries of truth because they sense the emptiness of many of our words; they can see the gap between what we say and what we live.[17]

No community can be self-correcting in principle. Criticism is possible only when there are those present who constitute a critical edge. Vanier, whose own presence for l'Arche creates a problem just to the extent some may think l'Arche depends on him, is surely right to suggest that communities like l'Arche at least have some purchase of being truthful to the extent they understand that truth often is spoken by those who cannot speak.[18]

Such communities are by necessity constituted by the practice of hospitality. This is not always easy, given Vanier's understanding of community as a grouping of people "who have left their own milieu to live with others under the same roof, and work from a new vision of human beings and their relationships with each other and with God."[19] Such communities can easily become ingrown and protective, but for a community that has learned to live with people with mental retardation, such protectiveness can only be destructive. The crucial question is not whether people are to be welcomed, but who is to make the decision who is to be welcomed and how. According to Vanier, in l'Arche communities those best able to discern who should be welcomed are people with mental retardation. "They have been in the community for a long time, often for longer than the assistants, and sometimes longer than the person in charge. It is important to consult these handicapped people before we welcome someone in distress."[20]

I am never sure how to characterize Vanier's observations about l'Arche. It seems right, however, that most of what he has to tell us takes the form of aphorisms — that is, short bursts of hard won wisdom not easily systemized or brought to a point. Wisdom is constituted by judgements about matters that matter. Yet to be wise requires we be part of traditions that form people like Vanier who can say what we all might see or experience, but lack the ability to say what we see. In short, if Vanier had not spent years living with people with mental retardation he would not have acquired the skills to now speak with and for them.

The wisdom that he shares with us, gentle though it be, cannot help but disrupt our lives. We read Vanier because we want to know how to do, if not be, good; but in knowing how to do good, we also discover that the subject is not people with mental retardation but us. For the great shock for many of us who want to be of help to people with mental retardation, because we think they are weak, is to discover our own weakness. As Vanier observes,

> It is always easier to accept the weakness of handicapped people — we are there precisely because we expect it — than our own weakness that often takes us by surprise! We want to see only good qualities in ourselves and other assistants. Growth begins when we start to accept our own weakness.[21]

What, moreover, could be more threatening for the handicapped than for them to expose our own sense of helplessness and loneliness?

To be able to be with people with mental retardation without being "helpful" is what l'Arche is about. It is slow work. Indeed, to be capable of such work means, as Vanier puts it, we have "to be great friends of time."[22] We have to become not only friends of time, but friends of those who make such time possible. And to make such time possible is to call upon One who, though outside of time, has entered into our time to be with us and to befriend us. We have to learn how to receive the friendship of people with mental retardation offer to us.

> When friendship encourages fidelity, it is the most beautiful thing of all. Aristotle calls it the flower of virtue; it has the gratuity of the flower. On the dark days, we need the refuge of friendship. When we feel flat or fed up, a letter from a friend can bring back peace and confidence. The Holy Spirit uses small things to comfort and strengthen us.[23]

Our care of people with mental retardation and their care of us is in the small things we do for one another. "Community is made of the gentle concern that people show each other every day. It is made of small gestures, of services and sacrifices which say 'I love you' and 'I'm happy to be with you'."[24] Vanier confesses that when he feels tired he goes to La Forestière. La Forestière is a house in his community where none of the nine or so people who live there can talk and most cannot walk. They must express their hearts and emotions through their bodies. The assistants at La Forestiere cannot work at their rhythm, but at that of the handicapped.

> Things have to go at a pace which can welcome their least expression; because they have no verbal skills, they have no way of enforcing their views by raising their voice. So the assistants have to be the more attentive to the many non-verbal communications, and this adds greatly to their ability to welcome the whole person. They become increasingly people of welcome and compassion. The slower rhythm and even the presence of the handicapped people makes me slow down, switch off my efficiency motor, rest and recognize the presence of God. The poorest people have an extraordinary power to heal the wounds in our hearts. If we welcome them, they nourish us.[25]

We, that is those of us external to the world of l'Arche communities, are tempted to characterize their work in heroic terms. But that is not how they understand what they do. As Vanier observes, love does not mean doing extraordinary things, but rather knowing how to do ordinary things with tenderness. He calls our attention to the significance of Jesus' "hidden life" — the thirty years he spent in Nazareth when no one knew he was the son of God. He lived family and community life in humility working with wood and having his life constituted by the small happenings of such a village. Jesus' hidden life is the model for all community life.[26] In his life we are given the time to be friends of the timeful friends we call people with mental retardation.

5. DOING THINGS WITH VANIER

To call attention to Vanier's witness is dangerous just to the extent it is so powerful. He and his friends' presence is too strong for most of us. We cannot imagine reproducing his work in our lives. It requires too much time, it requires too much "labour intensive involvement", it requires people willing to have their lives turned inside out, it assumes that what Christians believe about the world is true and can be lived. For many such requirements and assumptions seem utopian.

Yet they cannot be utopian because l'Arche communities exist. No doubt those in l'Arche often are less than they would wish, but that such a wish forms their desires indicates that they do not think they are pursuing some unrealizable ideal. Moreover, their witness remains crucial for the rest of us who are not part of their community; for without such examples our imaginations lack the resources to know that what we have become used to doing is not done by necessity. Without l'Arche anything I or any other theologian might have to say could not help but be empty. L'Arche literally gives weight, gives body, to the story of the world which Christians know as Gospel.

Because Vanier and his friends are so embodied by and in the story of Christ, they feel no need to give meaning to the lives of people with mental retardation. They feel no need to justify the care they give to people with mental retardation. They do not think they need to justify their "use" of people with mental retardation. Such questions and problems do not arise because you do not need to ask such questions about your friends. Friends need no justification. Friendship is a gift and, like most significant gifts, it is surrounded by mystery. We finally cannot explain friendship anymore than we can explain our existence. We can only delight in our friends.

Without such delight our care of people with mental retardation cannot help but seem pointless. Without delight the professional skills we gain to try to help people with mental retardation can too quickly become part of a mechanistic world of control. Vanier and his friends are certainly not disdainful of the wonderful technologies that have been developed to help people with handicaps.[27] Rather they see that such technologies can too easily become ends in themselves no longer serving friendship.

Yet is all this finally just "too Christian"? Vanier, after all, is obviously a person shaped by Catholic practice and thought.[28] How can what is learned in l'Arche be possible in a secular and pluralist world? I do not know for sure how Vanier would answer, but I suspect his answer might be something like this. What is possible in l'Arche is possible anywhere we find people willing to learn to live with people with mental retardation. After all, the God that is celebrated in l'Arche is God. Such a God knows no boundaries. If such a God can make people with mental retardation claim some of us as friends, surely such a God will be found among those who know not God. That such is the case after all is why what Christians believe about the world is called "good news". For is it not wonderful to discover in a world as terrible as this that God has created the time, given us friends of time in time, so that we might learn to be friends with one another and, yes, even God.

NOTES

1 J. Vanier, *Community and Growth*. London: Darton, Longman, and Todd, 1979, p. 3.
2 *Ibid.*, p. 80.
3 *Ibid.*, p. 106.
4 M. Berube, *Life As We Know It: A Father, a Family, and an Exceptional Child*. New York: Pantheon Books, 1996, p. 248. Berube may not appreciate the considerable differences between the accounts of justice by Rawls and Habermas but I think he rightly intuits that such differences in the face of people with mental retardation do not amount to much.
5 *Ibid.*, p. 247.
6 *Ibid.*, p. 47.
7 *Ibid.*, p. 48.
8 *Ibid.*, p. 264.
9 For my reflections on these matters see my *Naming the Silences: God, Medicine, and the Problem of Suffering*. Grand Rapids: Eerdmans, 1990. The second edition of the book was retitled as *God, Medicine, and Suffering*.
10 I. Kant, *Foundations of the Metaphysics of Morals*, tr. Lewis White Beck. New York: Liberal Arts Press, 1959, p. 47.
11 It is important to note that Kant quite sensibly assumed that it is sometimes permissible to treat people as means. What the imperative excludes is that treatment as a means occludes their status as ends. Of course this but creates the problem of how we are to know when someone has ever been treated as a "means only".
12 Berube, p. 112.
13 *Ibid.*, p. 113. Berube observes that what saves the unavoidability of Jamie being a subject is they as parents have the benefit of seeing Jamie's agents face to face. "They *are* agents: they are defined by their agency (in both senses), and Jamie is their agentless object, the name repeated a thousand times in the eight-inch stack of medical prognoses, cognitive evaluations, and assorted therapy reports that constitute the subject known as Jamie Lyon Berube. But they also happen to be our neighbours and friends. Rita Huddle, Jamie's first speech therapist at DSC, is also the mother of two of Nick's friends in a tae kwon do class, where we run into her regularly; Nancy Yeagle, his first occupational therapist, is also the mother of one of his playmates at day care as well as the spouse of the chef at a local Italian restaurant Jamie's quite fond of. And Sara Jane Annin, his case worker, is not only a friend and confidante, but the mother of *two* children with Down Syndrome", pp. 113-4.
14 This question is the title of Wendell Berry's wonderful book, *What Are People For?* San Francisco: North Point Press, 1990. The essay in the book that bears this title concerns the view by the "governing agricultural doctrine" of the government, universities, and corporations that there are too many people on the farm. Berry argues that this doctrine continues to be held even though the migration of people from the farms hurts the land and the cities. Yet "the great question that hovers over this issue, one that we have dealt with mainly by indifference, is the question of what people are *for*. Is their greatest dignity in unemployment? Is the obsolescence of human beings now our social goal? One would conclude so from our attitude toward work, especially the manual work necessary to the long-term preservation of the land, and from our rush toward mechanization, automation, and computerization. In a country that puts an absolute premium on labour-saving measures, short workdays, and retirement, why should there be any surprise at permanence of unemployment and welfare dependency? Those are only different names for our national ambitions." p. 12.
15 A. MacIntyre, *After Virtue*, Second Edition. Notre Dame: University of Notre Dame Press, 1984, p. 52. MacIntyre observes that Kant in the second book of the second *Critique* does acknowledge that a teleological framework is necessary for his ethics to be intelligible. (p. 56) The teleology Kant presumed was, of course, anthropocentric, not theocentric.

16 Put metaphysically, the practices that constitute l'Arche rightly assume that being is prior to knowing. Questions about what "meaning" people with mental retardation may or may not have are questions shaped by habits that assume the priority of epistemological questions. Berube's "now that he is here" reveals that the priorities of being cannot be repressed. I am indebted to Dr. Brett Webb-Mitchell for calling my attention to this connection.

17 Vanier, p. 200.

18 One cannot help but think Vanier is thinking about his own role in l'Arche when he observes, "I am sometimes a bit worried by communities which are carried by a single strong shepherd or a solidly united team of shepherds. As these communities have no traditions, no history and no constitutional control by a recognized legal authority, there is hardly any check on their activities. The leaders may develop a taste for their role, seeing themselves as indispensable, and so unconsciously dominating others. There is also the risk of mixing community and spiritual power. It is good and useful if these spiritual shepherds quickly hand over direction of the community to someone else, so that they can be freer to exercise their gift of priest and shepherd." Vanier, p. 176. He observes he is concerned about communities without any traditions who refuse to accept external authority. They will not outlive their founder for long and, if there is no external control, the founder will be in danger of making some serious mistakes. (p. 86.)

19 *Ibid.*, p. 2.

20 *Ibid.*, p. 197. Vanier observes that to welcome is not primarily to open the doors of our house, but to open our hearts by becoming vulnerable.

21 *Ibid.*, p. 88.

22 *Ibid.*, p. 80.

23 *Ibid.*, p. 135. Vanier's remarks on friendship are particularly interesting given his philosophical training. He wrote his dissertation at the Institut Catholique in Paris on Aristotle's ethics. He knows well that for Aristotle character friendship would be impossible between those thought to be "normal" and the "handicapped". One cannot help but think that Vanier's life exemplifies how Aquinas' contention that the goal of life is to be befriended by God explodes Aristotle's understanding of friendship. I am indebted to Brett Webb-Mitchell's account of Vanier as well as his study of l'Arche in his *L'Arche: An Ethnographic Study of persons with Disabilities Living in a Community with Non-Disabled People*. Ph.D Dissertation: University of North Carolina, 1988. Since writing his dissertation, Webb-Mitchell has published a series of books that explore the theological significance of people with mental retardation and, in particular, how friendship with them is possible. See his *God Plays Piano, Too*. New York: Crossroads, 1993; *Unexpected Guests at God's Banquet*. New York: Crossroads, 1994; and *Dancing with Disabilities*. Cleveland: United Church Press, 1996.

24 Vanier, p. 26.

25 *Ibid.*, p. 139-140.

26 *Ibid.*, p. 220.

27 *Ibid.*, p. 106.

28 Vanier observes, "As I think of all the communities throughout the world, struggling for growth, yearning to answer the call of Jesus and of the poor, I realize the need for a universal shepherd, a shepherd who yearns for unity, who has clarity of vision, who calls forth communities and who holds all people. I was deeply touched by the election of John-Paul I and even more touched by the election of John-Paul II. How long will it take before people realize this deep need? How long will it take for Catholics to understand the depths of their gifts and to be confounded in humility? How long will it take Catholics to recognize the beauty and gift in the Protestant churches, especially their love of Scripture and of announcing the Word? And one day will Protestant churches discover the immensity of riches hidden in the Eucharist? Yes, I yearn for this day." (p. 104).

PIETER A. DE RUYTER

CHAPTER 11

EXPERIENCE OF MEANING IN HUMAN ENCOUNTER

1. INTRODUCTION

The meaning of the life of people with mental retardation is experienced in the encounter, in an openness to their unique person, in the readiness to give *and* receive, in a sincere concern for their well-being. In this chapter, I wish to develop this thesis by means of addressing four questions:

- What turns a contact between two people into an encounter?
- What are the obstacles that prevent us from encountering people with mental retardation?
- How can, in spite of these obstacles, an encounter come about?
- How can one experience the meaning of (the other's and his own) life in such an encounter?

2. NOT EVERY CONTACT IS AN ENCOUNTER

The word "encounter" tends to be used in season and out of season. All too easy do people say that they have encountered each other, when in reality they had only a brief and superficial exchange. By these kinds of statements, the meaning of the concept loses its substance. For this reason, I will use the term "encounter" in a specific way. A human encounter always takes place unexpectedly. One cannot arrange to have an encounter. An encounter always has a strong personal character. People who encounter one another are open-minded, honest, and ready to give and receive. An encounter does not leave the participant unaffected. It is coupled with strong emotions; the person is delighted, saddened, shocked, or agitated. An encounter causes someone to stop and think. It leads him to the meaning of his life, to the things that really matter to him.

When using the concept in this fashion, it is clear that a human encounter is not a daily occurrence. Without encounters, a life would be superficial, but too many encounters would be overtaxing. Too many thoughts directed toward oneself in relation to others will hamper one's daily functioning and take away all spontaneity. Still, although one cannot arrange to have an encounter in this sense, there are a

Joop Stolk, Theo A. Boer & Ruth Seldenrijk (eds.). Meaningful Care, 155—165

number of conditions one must answer in order to make an encounter possible. First of all, there must be *a purposeful contact* with clear expectations. When meeting another person, one normally aims for something. One expects something from the contact. Only when one wants something with, from, or for the other person, can an encounter take place. Simply sitting next to someone in the bus, for example, is not yet an encounter. Agreeing to travel to work together on the bus creates the possibility for an encounter, especially when this intention is coupled with the expectation that you will enjoy each other's company.

The second condition is *susceptibility*. One has to be open to the possibility that an encounter with someone else might cause us to see things in a new perspective. An encounter cannot occur when one's mind is set only on one's own goals. This closed attitude makes it impossible for someone to receive something new, especially if it is radically new. When professionals have a closed-minded approach to their work with people with mental retardation, they will only reinforce the truth of their own thinking, and will shut out any opportunity for having an encounter. He who wants to encounter someone, must be open to the input of this other person.

The third and most important condition is *interdependence*. An encounter with another person is experienced most deeply when one realizes that one person cannot live without the other. He who positions himself exclusively as the giving, caring, and helping party in his contact with people with mental retardation, shuts out any possibility of having an encounter. He who encounters another person, gives and receives with the realization that the other is indispensable.

People can encounter one another in different ways, under various circumstances, and with variable intentions. One encounter is different from the next. In making a differentiation, I assume there to be a tight connection between human actions and the manner in which encounters take place. In this context, three types of actions can be identified:

Defensive Actions — People act defensively when they feel threatened by something or someone. The primary intent of their actions is to "survive".

Enterprising Actions — This stems from the human desire for self-realization. The primary intent of these actions is to "acquire".

Responsive Actions — People act in response to an appeal made by someone else. The primary intent of these kinds of actions is to "affirm" the other.

In connection to these actions, three types of encounters can be identified:

Encounter as intruding into my defensive actions

Suppose that I feel threatened by someone, perhaps by his words, or perhaps by his actions. When I react in a defensive manner, the other could respond with a look or a word that could cause me to become flustered. By this look, or word, the other intrudes into my survival strategy. He might, for example, ask me, "why this superior behaviour? Why do you attempt to belittle me?" I get confused, feel ashamed, and wonder whether my behaviour was justified. It is also possible that the other asks, "why do you defend yourself? Am I that dangerous; isn't your fear out of place?" Such a break-through actually could free me from my assumption that I must defend myself. As stated before, encounters are characterized by self-reflection and strong emotions. This does not mean that an encounter will always lead me to change my behaviour. I could, for example, drown out any shame I feel about my uncalled for behaviour by becoming even more defensive. This will put an end to the encounter.

Encounter as a discovery correcting my enterprising actions
Suppose that, in a contact with someone, I intend to gain knowledge for myself, receive affection from the other, or gain control over the other. I purposely invest much time and energy in this contact. Suppose now, that the other becomes aware of my intentions and does not accept this. He confronts me with my doublemindedness, and sees right through my intentions. My enterprising actions turn into a discovery. I discover that I am short-changing the other person with the way I am acting. For example, I develop a treatment plan for a woman with mental retardation. When putting the plan into action, I discover that I have been too hasty with my assumptions on several important points. Through her protests, the woman brings to my realization the fact that I was trying to put her into a box. I am embarrassed because I did not take her individuality into account. I also might be very surprised by her input; I now need to drastically change the treatment plan. I have to admit that she differs completely from the way I had pictured her. Through my encounter with people with mental retardation, I realize that my involvement should have taken the form of a dialogue rather than simply following a recipe. The encounter has the character of a discovery.

Encounter as an act of grace in answer to my responsive actions
Suppose that someone asks me for help, and I decide to respond. I help him, support him, and give him what he needs. In short, I am there for him without reserve. It is not guaranteed, however, that my response is the answer to what the other asks of me. Even with the best intentions, I might act wrongfully because, for instance, I did not listen well enough to the other person. This often happens when adults raise children. Even before the child has finished his question, I, the adult, know what he is asking; at least, I think I know. The child however, is not served by my answer and makes that clear to me, and I end up feeling ashamed for my poor listening skills. However, the child makes clear that, although I understood him wrongly, he knows my intentions were good. The child does not judge me. He gives me the opportunity to try again. In doing so, the encounter with the child has the nature of an act of grace. Such meetings are invaluable. The contact with the child is left free of any obligation, and the adult is grateful. He experiences the encounter with the child as a gift: "who am I, to be treated this way?" Such an experience frees up new energy, vital energy, and keeps the adult going for a while.

3. OBSTACLES TO THE ENCOUNTER

Being confronted with people who have mental retardation calls up intense feelings.

Receiving the news that their child is mentally handicapped can bring on a time of crisis for parents. The first experiences of working with people with mental retardation can be so upsetting for health care providers, that they might come to doubt whether they chose the right profession.

Although I mentioned earlier that an encounter is coupled with strong emotions, the emotion that is coupled with this confrontation with people with mental retardation should not be assumed to be the result of an encounter. This emotion usually does not come about by being confronted with a person with mental retardation, but through being confronted with his or her handicaps. This confrontation tends to be more a threat to, rather than the beginning of, an encounter.

The fact that a confrontation can become a threat to a real encounter stems from the fact that people are natural and cultural beings. By nature, a human being protects himself against everything that threatens his survival. When experiencing something dangerous, he instinctively tries to escape from the danger. Knowing that something strange could be dangerous, he tries to keep this "strangeness" at a distance. He who sees a person with a serious mental handicap, is startled and shrinks back. The other is experienced to be repulsive.

Where does this aversion come from? As humans, we tend to have an image of the ideal person. In our culture, two images of the ideal person dominate. The first picture consists of the elements, "young, intelligent, verbal, and social." The successful person is the star in show-business, the brilliant scientist, the dynamic politician, and the enterprising business-man. The second picture of the ideal person came into existence in reaction to the first one. It is the flip-side of the first picture: self-actualization rather than adapting to others, autonomy rather than sensitivity toward other's wishes, and being critical of a consumptive and material world.

No matter if we compare a person with mental retardation to the first or to the second image, he will always fall short. He will never be able to answer to the ideals and idols of our culture. We always view people with mental retardation out of our culturally determined biases. This is also true for those who have a profession dealing with the care for people with mental retardation.

It is characteristic of professional care-givers to interact with their clients and patients on basis of their specialized learning and skills. Through their learning and skills, they have developed a specialistic view of people. This is inherent to their profession, and therefore unavoidable. There is a danger, however, that the care-giver selects all his information on this basis. Whatever he sees, hears, and experiences, he fits into his professional viewpoint. He slices away, as it were, those facets of his clients with mental retardation that do not fit his image. When the image he has formed rests on scientific research based on a statistical normality model, or on an aristocratic model, the person with mental retardation becomes an aberration of the norm, a threat to the ideal image. If this image becomes part and parcel of his care-giving strategy, the person with mental retardation is reduced to a person with a shortcoming, missing something he has yet to obtain. As a result, the care provider becomes the giver, and the person with the mental handicap the receiver. These fixed roles are a serious obstacle to the encounter. Is it possible that they would even prevent the occurrence of an encounter?

4. ENCOUNTERS WITH PEOPLE WITH MENTAL RETARDATION

In order to get an answer to the question whether fixed roles could prevent the occurrence of an encounter, I approached several group leaders and pedagogic counsellors involved in the care of people with mental retardation. I requested them to relate a personal experience that made them stop and think. In their work with people with mental retardation, what event had they never forgotten? I then asked them to recall how this experience helped them come, or continue, to view this resident as a unique person.

Twenty-eight group leaders responded. I interpreted their stories on basis of the aforementioned characteristics of the encounter, and then divided them into the three types of encounters: intruding into defensive actions, correcting enterprising actions, and an act of grace in answer to responsive actions. As an illustration, I will briefly relate three stories of each type of encounter, followed by some side remarks. It needs to be said that these stories should not be read as "success-stories". In the context of care of people with mental retardation, the possibilities of having true human encounters are limited. It is my contention, however, that these limits are not fixed. When group leaders and parents, despite all their efforts, do not succeed in passing these limits, this is not a matter of fault, but of powerlessness. This powerlessless should motivate counsellors to help parents and group leaders to find possible ways to have encounters with people with mental retardation.

4.1. Encounter as Intruding into the Defensive Actions of the Care-giver

"Carey"

Carey, a girl with a mild mental handicap who is eighteen years old, is known to be "difficult". She is often aggressive, and as a result frequently breaks objects in and around the home. In the house where she lives, both residents and care-givers are afraid of her. One day, Carey has another eruption of anger. Anything she finds near her, she throws through the room. No one is able to calm her down. Just as Carey is starting to hit a group leader, a colleague, who is standing nearby, jumps in to help. Together, they try to subdue Carey. They pull her out of the living room and into the bathroom. Carey screams and yells. The group leader wets her face and talks with her in a soft tone of voice. Suddenly, Carey slumps down, and calls out, "oh, I am so bad!" The group leader responds, "no, you're not; you just *feel* bad." Carey starts crying with intense sadness. The group leader sits down next to her on the ground. Carey leans up against her, and says, "please hold me; hold me tight." For the group leader, the image of the difficult, unapproachable girl is broken. Carey seeks safety. Afterwards, the group leader does not understand why she never saw that before.

"Daniel"

A group leader is regularly at odds with Daniel, a boy with mental retardation, sixteen years of age. He considers Daniel stubborn, contrary, and unruly. One day, Daniel refuses to take off his shoes in the gym, and the group leader confronts him and really gives it to him. Daniel should do what he is told. A little later, he notices that Daniel has wet his pants. "He did that to spite me," thinks the group leader, and he heads for Daniel to inform him that he does not accept such behaviour. When he nears Daniel, he notices that the boy has scratches on his arms and face. Out of fear for a fellow resident, who threatened him, Daniel has urinated in his pants. The group leader writes, "I was deeply embarrassed, and from that moment on, I looked at him differently. With Daniel, I can now see the difference between him having his own will, and being wilful."

"Ellen"
It is not easy to establish contact with Ellen, a forty year old woman. The little contact there is usually takes place in connection with her difficult behaviour. She takes food away from other residents, and smears her stool. During a bus ride, Ellen sits next to Betty, a resident who does not feel comfortable on the bus. The comfort and reassurance given by the staff does not seem to help. Ellen, in turn, is affected, and starts looking sadder by the minute. At one point, she puts her hand on the leg of her partner in distress, and begins stroking it. For a short moment, Betty stops crying, but when she starts crying again, Ellen takes her hand and cries with her. The staff is very impressed, because no one had expected such behaviour from Ellen. The group leader writes, "that event greatly affected my feelings, expectations, and attitude toward Ellen. She became a completely different person."

In these three stories, the contact between the group leaders and residents takes on the character of an encounter. At first, the contact is mostly considered burdensome. Then, something unexpected happens, something that does not fit the image held of this person by the group leaders. The aggressive Carey asks to be held. The once thought-to-be spiteful Daniel asks for protection. The socially inept Ellen shares in Betty's sorrow.

Out of these three stories, it becomes apparent how significant it is to be open to the new. It would have been tempting to continue bringing Carey to the bathroom to cool down each time she got upset, to tell Daniel that it is for his own good and that for a change he can feel how he always makes others feel, and to be patronizing toward Ellen, telling each other that she's becoming sentimental. But this was not how the contact ended. The group leaders were susceptible to the unexpected. The reaction of the residents affected them; they allowed themselves to be influenced.

A repeated theme in the stories is the shame felt by the group leaders about a previous bias they had held, or about their lack of open-mindedness. The writers realize that they damaged the integrity of the resident. In two stories, the staff demonstrates a natural aversion toward the resident with mental retardation. They are afraid of Carey's aggression, and Ellen is dirty, because she smears her stool. It also is of note how the professional character of the interaction is a threat to the encounter. The professional appears to have a fixed image of the resident. He thinks he understands the resident, and on this ground thinks he knows how to interact with the resident. Daniel is wilful and Ellen is socially inept. The professionals have a way of dealing with both issues; fitting in with the picture they have formed of the resident, they act routinely. Yet, through the encounter, the group leader (re)discovers that the resident has, as a person, the right to be accepted just as he is and just as he acts. He has the right to be recognized as an individual.

Finally, we read how the encounter changes the attitude and actions of the group leaders. They notice Carey's need for safety. Daniel's group leader becomes more open-minded, and after the day trip, Ellen is looked at with different eyes.

4.2. Encounter as a Discovery which Crosses through Enterprising Actions

"Peter"
Peter is a 10 year old boy with mental retardation who is temporarily living on an observation unit. At present, there are nine other children in the group, younger than him, and functioning at a much lower level. The members of staff view him as one of the ten. The same rules count for him as for the other children. The doors are locked, all the children go to bed at the same time, they play in a closed area, etc. Peter starts to rebel. In the mind of the group leaders, he is a difficult child. But after some time, they start wondering whether Peter's resistance is characteristic of him, or whether it is related to his situation. The question is difficult to answer until, after a heavy conflict, Peter indicates what is bothering him: "you guys treat me like a child, I'm not crazy!" The staff can't deny his accusations. They realize how they have short-changed Peter. As a result, they decide to radically change their behaviour toward Peter. Peter receives a key to the front door, he is allowed to stay up later than the other children, and he may ride his bike outside of the closed area.

"Coby"
Coby is a woman with mental retardation. She is not able to speak, and is not able to use sign language. At age twenty-three, she moves from her home to a group home for young adults with mental retardation. After only a few weeks of staying there, she is transferred to another residence, without being given a reason. Within a few weeks after the transfer, she starts banging her head and opens up a small wound by scratching. In order to prevent her from hurting herself more, her wrists are restrained. Now she begins biting her lower lip, which becomes a large bleeding wound. She refuses to eat. This continues for several weeks. The staff is at a loss what to do. Then, the head of the department decides to take on a radically different approach. Coby's restraints are removed, and she receives a personal attendant. When needed, this attendant uses her own hands to protect Coby from her self-mutilating behaviour. She often sings and makes music with Coby. Within only a few days, assistance is no longer needed at night. Coby starts eating again, and when she is a little stronger, she moves back to the first residence. Now, she is once again the cheerful, active, and resilient woman that she was during the first weeks of her stay there. The group leader writes, "this event was a shocking experience for me. We waltzed right over her. It never occurred to us that she did not want to be transferred. We left her with only one option: to sound the alarm by hurting herself.

Had we taken her wishes into account, and interpreted her self-mutilating behaviour correctly, this miserable situation would never have come to pass."

"Walter"
When a pedagogic counsellor begins his work in a residential facility, he "inherits" a sixty-four year old man, whose file describes him as having mental retardation, with serious spasticity, hospital-dependent, and with a maximum care need. During the first weeks, they have little contact, nothing more than a greeting when they see each other in the hallway. After a month, the pedagogic counsellor decides to establish contact with Walter. When he enters his little room, Walter asks him to wait because Tsjaikowsky's 6th symphony is still playing. The counsellor writes, "I was really moved, perhaps because of my personal love for music, but probably more because of how he asked me. I marvelled at his reaction; it was a surprise to me. I tried talking to him about music. Although it was with difficulty, we understood each other. With time, I came to know him better, and he seemed to blossom. I discovered that the issue wasn't so much that he was hospital dependent, but rather that his spirit had, as it were, been broken by the restrictive system." The pedagogic counsellor now takes Walter's individuality into account as much as he can. He takes him to concerts, shops for c.d.'s with him, and makes sure that his privacy is respected.

The tie that binds these stories is that the care-givers here act in a way that suits them best. It is easier, after all, if Peter is one of ten, if Coby is satisfied with her transfer, and if the contact with Walter takes place when it fits into the pedagogic counsellor's schedule. But Peter, Coby, and Walter protest against how their care-givers acted out of self-interest, without taking part in a dialogue with them. Their reaction reveals how the care-giver only seeks his own interests, and that this hurts them (sometimes literally). Since they do not put up with this, an encounter occurs.

In the stories of Peter and Coby, the encounter arises in a similar fashion. Peter and Coby are forced to give clearer and clearer signals. Coby even has to go to the extreme, hurting herself in order to show her care-givers what they are doing to her. Walter's story is different. Walter has to wait years before having an encounter with a care-giver, and even then he is lucky that this is someone who also loves music.

What the stories have in common is that the residents need to give a strong signal. It is only in this manner that the care-givers are jolted enough to be illuminated about the uniqueness of the residents. The fact that it takes so long is, in my opinion, related to the intentions of the care-givers. They want to reach a certain goal, and interpret resistance as being the resident's problem. Only when a clear signal is given, does the care-giver re-orient himself. He is startled, and realizes that he has put this person in a box.

These stories again bring to light how important it is for care-givers to be susceptible to new input, not to keep interpreting Peter's protests as resistance, or continuing to put even more restrictions on Coby in response to her behaviour. Being susceptible to new input means to not ignore Walter's order to wait, and to not smile at the thought that Walter is trying to give the impression that he likes music, but to wait to be let into the room, and to take him seriously.

If, by correcting the enterprising actions of the care-giver, an encounter takes place, the emotion is stronger than would be the case if the care-giver were to break through the defensive behaviour of the resident. The care-giver knows he is without excuse. He failed and is guilty. He has reduced the resident into an object. This also explains the radical change in the actions of the care-givers. Peter's group leaders give him his own key and let him go into town by himself. They stick to these measures, even when their colleagues have negative reactions. Coby goes back to the home where she seemed to feel safe, and Walter is truly respected as a music lover.

Why does it take so long for the care-givers to have an encounter with Peter, Coby, and Walter? The writers themselves explain their failing as a sort of professional deformity. Peter's group leader writes, "until that moment, someone with mental retardation was simply a dependent person, lacking his own identity." The writer of Coby's story remarks that at Coby's first negative reactions, they immediately fell back on using well-known therapeutic strategies for handling self-mutilating behaviour, without asking themselves why Coby was reacting this way. Finally, the writer of Walter's story points out that he had fully accepted the image described in Walter's file, which led him to consider Walter to be a man who is handicapped in every respect.

Through unexpected encounters with people with mental retardation, the care-giver (re)discovers that the people in question are their own unique person who have a great deal to tell and offer. He becomes aware of the risk of merely acting as care-giver. An encounter requires the involvement of the whole person.

4.3. Encounter as an Act of Grace in Reaction to the Responsive Actions of the Staff

"Jack"

A group leader writes about Jack, an eight year old boy, who is autistic and who has a mental handicap. In many different ways, she attempts to involve Jack with the world of people. But Jack does not seem to have a need for this. He shuns all contact. He has never even had eye-contact with her. But the group leader does not give up, and continues to think of ways to reach him. Unfortunately, she has little success. Then, one day, Jack happens to sit down next to her, and she quietly starts singing a song. By means of gesturing, Jack makes clear to her that he wants her to continue singing. This was far beyond anyone's expectations. During the weeks that follow, Jack regularly sits down by her, and then points at his own mouth and at her mouth. This is a signal to the group leader that she should sing with him. During the singing, Jack sits close to the group leader, but does not want to be touched. He resists her putting an arm around his shoulder. Yet, it is still a great gain. Jack's bubble of isolation has been burst. The group leader considers it a privilege that Jack has allowed her into his world.

"Annie"

Annie is a girl with mental retardation who is nine years old. She was placed out of the home when she was a baby, and has lived in a residential facility ever since. She never goes home and is rarely visited. The group leader regularly takes Annie home with her. This, of course, is beyond her call of duty, but Annie really enjoys being with the family, and the little things that are taken for granted by the average person are very special to her. She enjoys going to the grocery store, picking out vegetables, snacks, and drinks. She helps with meal preparation, and decorates the dinner table with a flower or a candle. Annie does all this with a level of enthusiasm that continues to amaze the group leader. This is not how she knows Annie. What started as an obligation, grew into a series of encounters which brought the group leader great enjoyment. Because of Annie, the group leader's eyes were opened to the special things in ordinary daily life.

"Nowse, big nowse!"

A pedagogic counsellor writes about an encounter that happened a long time ago: "a mentally handicapped man comes leaping towards me to meet me, waving with his arms. He enthusiastically shouts, 'nowse, nowse, big nowse!' His face radiates, 'nowse, nowse, big nowse!' He stops right in front of me, jumps up and down a few times, and then squeezes my nose between his thumb and index finger. I have the urge to push him away, but I control myself. I don't want to think about his dirty fingers, or the bad breath coming from his mouth. I focus only on his face, which radiates with enthusiasm, 'nowse, nowse, big nowse!' He is excited about what I wouldn't exactly call my most attractive body part. But what does this man know about my negative feelings regarding my big nose? He thinks it's magnificent and, in an incredible way, he manages to cause me to share in his joy. It may sound crazy, but we were rolling in laughter."

These examples demonstrate that an "encounter as an act of grace" does not have an exclusive character (as the choice of words would have us assume), but rather is a part of ordinary, every day life. A group leader sings with an autistic boy. Another group leader goes shopping, cooks dinner, and sits at a decorated table with her little guest. A pedagogic counsellor bumps into a man with mental retardation on the street, and they have fun together. It could not get more ordinary. Nothing unusual happens. Three professionals, who have been trained to provide help, are helped themselves. This is how Jack's group leader learns to pick up on the way in which an autistic child wants to encounter her, this is how Annie's group leader is taught to experience joy in the little things, and this is how the pedagogic counsellor learns to laugh about her big nose.

Those who work with people with mental retardation, have learned to take initiative, to stimulate, and to look for new and creative ideas to reach people who can be difficult to understand, show little initiative, and tend to give up at the first set-back. What these three examples have in common is that the tables are turned. The professional has to learn to let another take the initiative, to be prepared to be stimulated by another person, and to never give up. This does not happen automatically, as the examples show.

Jack's group leader follows a prescribed regimen said to stimulate the social development of autistic children, but discovers that it doesn't work in this case. She learns to have an eye for the unexpected and to take into account Jack's "regimen": singing together, but only at specific moments; sitting close together, but without touching.

Annie's group leader feels sorry for a child who does not know what family life is like, and who has nearly no one who cares enough about her to visit. The group leader feels obliged to break through Annie's isolation. She does what can be expected from a group leader: she brings the child into a normal family, and broadens her experience by having her join in the daily chores. And then, the contact with the "lonely mentally handicapped child" becomes an encounter. What once was work, now becomes life: sharing life with a child who ends up having a lot to offer her, such as community and cosiness. The group leader is no longer the benefactor of the child, but by an act of grace, ends up on the receiving end.

It is expected that a professional can maintain a balance between keeping distance and becoming personally involved. The pedagogic counsellor of the last example is put to the test in this regard. Will she stop the man from touching her nose in order to keep her distance, or will she allow this unknown mentally handicapped man to cross her personal boundaries. Professionals are taught to make a well considered choice, but the pedagogic counsellor does not choose. At first, she attempts to consciously control herself, but then she allows herself to be pulled along with the man's enthusiasm. This is even more remarkable, because he touches upon a sensitive area, which she would rather keep hidden. That, which she has never dared to face, happens in this encounter with a man with mental retardation. She allows herself to be seen as she really is. This is not her own achievement; it is a gift from another.

5. CLOSING REMARKS

The central theme in this book is the question about the meaning of care, particularly of the care of people with mental retardation. In this chapter, I argued that the meaning of a person's life is experienced in the encounter. I have developed this thesis by means of asking four questions: (1) how can a contact between persons turn into an encounter? (2) which obstacles can hinder the encounter with people who have mental retardation? (3) how can such an encounter as yet take place? and (4) how can a care-giver experience the fact that the life of people with mental retardation has meaning?

The latter two questions were answered by referring to nine stories of special encounters. They indicated that care-givers can experience meaning in the lives of people with mental retardation if they are willing to climb down from the ivory tower of their expertise, if they open their preconceived ideas to discussion, and set themselves up in a susceptible and dependent manner, full of expectation. He who has doubts about the meaning of life of a person with mental retardation, first should ask himself: have I ever truly encountered this child, this man, this woman?

JOOP STOLK

CHAPTER 12

EXPERIENCE OF MEANING IN DAILY CARE FOR PEOPLE WITH MENTAL RETARDATION

1. INTRODUCTION

When things go well, one doesn't usually wonder whether one's life, work, marriage, or parenting is meaningful. Questions about meaning usually come about when one experiences a fundamental deficiency. In their work, pedagogic counsellors[1] can get confronted with extreme situations, in which parents and children get completely stuck. Feelings of disappointment, sadness, and powerlessness predominate. People wonder if life this way holds any meaning. What value is there in continuing with each other under such circumstances?

This contribution will address the question of the meaning of care for people with mental retardation. By means of a case study, I will show how a pedagogic counsellor is confronted with the question of the meaning of his work. Based on this case study, I will present a few guidelines with which one can analyze crises in the experience of meaning of pedagogic counsellors (and like professionals). Finally, I will discuss the foundations of experiencing meaning. Under which conditions can the care of people with mental retardation be a meaningful experience?

2. "STUCK": A CASE STUDY

> For the past three years, Steven Hendriks (29 years old) has been working as a pedagogic counsellor for an institution that cares for people with mental retardation. It is his first job. He supports seven small-scale homes, spread out over a large area. He enjoys his work. He feels that he has something to offer. The group leaders also really appreciate him, particularly because his input is so practical. Two years ago, Steven got involved with the care of Frank who has the illness of Spielmeyer-Vogt. Because his vision declined rapidly over a short period of time, he was moved within the institution to "Westeinde", a home which is specialized in the care of children and youth with multiple (mental and visual) handicaps.
>
> The prognosis of children with the illness of Spielmeyer-Vogt is poor.

Joop Stolk, Theo A. Boer & Ruth Seldenrijk (eds.). Meaningful Care, 167—181

The illness is usually discovered at the age of six or eight, and is progressive, with the most important features being degeneration of the nervous system, development of spasticity and epilepsy, personality changes such as increased irritability, and declining mental abilities, vision, and speech. The poor vision is usually noted first. This was also the reason for Frank's transfer.

When Frank came to Westeinde, he was seven years old, and a cheerful boy. He paid little attention to his group-mates. His sole attention was toward the group leaders. At that time, he was already dependent on them for most things. Frank could not walk; he used his wheelchair to get around. His hearing was poor, and he could not speak. He communicated by use of a communication book (pointing to any of 35 drawn pictures in a notebook), and by using two hand signs: for "ready" and for "play". Together with the group leaders, the pedagogic counsellor developed a care plan which tuned into Frank's expected decline, particularly in view of his declining vision. The sighted symbols in his communication book were changed into tactile symbols with use of swell-paper. Similar practical solutions were arrived at for various other problems by means of close collaboration between the pedagogic counsellor and the group leaders.

For Frank's first year and a half at Westeinde, the pedagogic counsellor was closely involved with him. They had regular contact, at least once every two weeks, if not more. They would "talk", do something together (usually go for a walk), and afterwards Steven would have a meal with Frank and his group mates. If Frank was ill, Steven would call the group leaders to inquire about him.

During the last few months, Frank declined rapidly. His care became more custodial. Frank stayed in bed most of the day. His seizures increased in frequency and intensity. He rarely used his communication book, because holding it had become difficult, and because his mental abilities had greatly declined. This had its repercussions on the team, for everyone in their own way. The group leaders had a strong bond with Frank, and did all they could to lighten the serious effects of his illness. The pedagogic counsellor felt he was not needed any more. In his view, he had little to contribute to Frank's care. He slowly started distancing himself from Frank, as well as from the group leaders. He visited Westeinde less frequently, and when he did come, he felt he had nothing to offer. This did not mean that he wasn't thinking about Frank. On the contrary, he thought about him very much, especially when with his own family. Without intention, he compared Frank to his own children, who were active and full of life. He was filled with a sense of powerlessness in being of any meaning to Frank anymore. He had heard from a colleague how children with Spielmeyer-Vogt come to their end, and he often wished that it all was over.

Steven was not able to attend the last team conference on Frank's care plan. The group leaders resented this. They blamed him for pulling out of the "Frank case," and for also leaving the group leaders out in the cold. They were very disappointed: their teamwork had been so good, and then he just withdrew. This was not the Steven they knew. Their greatest grievance was that he had not come to see Frank for three whole months. Their accusations hit Steven very hard. He did not know how to respond except to say, "you are right."

3. CRISIS IN THE EXPERIENCE OF MEANING

The impasse in which the pedagogic counsellor found himself, can be typified as a crisis in the experience of meaning. The crisis had a history of two years. The pedagogic counsellor started out his work with Frank with enthusiasm. He loved working together with the group leaders on solving problems concerning a child with severe multiple disabilities, and on coming up with practical solutions. The time and energy put into carrying out the care plan were put to good use. It was meaningful and valuable work. This was apparent in the appreciation of the group leaders. It also was evident in Frank's functioning: for a year and a half he was helped by the carefully developed adjustments. But then Frank started regressing more rapidly. The pedagogic counsellor started doubting: was it possible to make a meaningful contribution to Frank's plan of care, now that he was less able, and now that his care-givers kept having to take steps backward? He noticed how the group leaders were focusing more on Frank's physical care. He considered that to be a task of the group leaders, to which he had little to contribute professionally. He pulled back from a situation which stood in sharp contrast to his private life. When he saw his own children, he was hit with doubts about the meaning of the life of a child like Frank, a child without a future. Since this was difficult to be confronted with, he avoided all contact with Frank. The group leaders interpreted his avoidance as disinterest. The pedagogic counsellor conceded, probably because at that moment, he was incapable of explaining how much the "Frank case" caused him to doubt the meaning of his professional work and the meaning of the lives of children such as Frank.

What could the pedagogic counsellor have done about this impasse? I see at least three possibilities. The first possibility is that he transfers the case to a colleague who can have a fresh look on things. This, however, would be the road of least resistance and for that reason not an attractive option. Moreover, it is very possible that such a transfer is not a possible option within his organization. A second possibility is that the pedagogic counsellor is amenable to the group leaders, pulls himself together, and picks up his work with renewed courage. This option does not hold up in actuality, however; for as experience teaches, in these sorts of situations, "new courage" does not last very long. A third possibility is that the pedagogic counsellor does not jump into action, but that he first reflects on the question of how he landed in this impasse, and of why he no longer finds meaning in his work. This is the most appropriate option for several reasons. A critical evaluation of one's own work and personal functioning provides needed clarity for the pedagogic counsellor as well as for the group leaders. This evaluation creates the possibility of breaking through the impasse and of re-orienting to his work from a solid foundation.

Next should be considered what this critical evaluation should focus on. What, in this case, are relevant focal points for the pedagogic counsellor in evaluating his work? The answer to this question requires a deeper understanding of the origin of his crisis in experiencing meaning. How did he reach a roadblock in the care of this child? For now, this is my answer: the crisis originated in the fact that, over the course of two years, the care of the pedagogic counsellor was decreasingly tuned into Frank's changing needs. As the child's dependence and physical care needs grew, the pedagogic counsellor increasingly doubted the meaning of his work, and the meaning of the child's life.

This "grand diagnosis" needs to be worked out in greater detail. I will do that in a stepwise fashion. First, I will (broadly) examine the conditions under which the work of a pedagogic counsellor can be considered "good". To do this, I will use the criteria for the quality of care, developed by De Ruyter.[2] Second, I will use these criteria to examine the actions of the pedagogic counsellor in the case study, and will indicate how his experience of meaning is influenced by his work-style.

4. CRITERIA FOR QUALITY

De Ruyter considers the work of a pedagogic counsellor to be good when it is done in a skilful, mutual, and authentic way. These three criteria are connected to the three dimensions found in human action: the technical, relational, and expressive dimensions.

First is the *technical* dimension. When a pedagogic counsellor provides guidance to a child (together with the group leaders), he has a goal in mind. This goal does not stand by itself. Ideally, the fulfillment of a goal (such making food choices) contributes to the realization of a larger ideal (such as guiding people with mental retardation toward optimal independence). Suppose that a pedagogic counsellor runs into an undesirable situation at work; for example, a child is being overtaxed. Then, identifying and interpreting the situation, formulating goals, choosing and acting on a course of action to improve the situation, are all elements of the technical dimension of human action. If the pedagogic counsellor masters these elements, he does his work skilfully. His skill is expressed in the way he plans, develops, executes, evaluates, and adjusts his treatment plans.

The *relational* dimension of human action pertains to the disposition of the pedagogic counsellor. His disposition is expressed in the manner in which he handles a child, and in how he thinks and talks about the child. This relational dimension is qualified with the criterion of mutuality. A pedagogic counsellor acts mutually, when he is able to balance the child's interests and his own interests and when he is able to build up trust with the child. A pedagogic counsellor who talks about a child in his or her presence, is not acting mutually. By such actions, a trusting relationship with the child is placed at risk. By talking over the child's head, he puts his desire to quickly discuss the "case" above the interests of the child. His actions do not meet the criterion of mutuality.

The technical and relational dimensions of human action concern relationships with other people. The third, *expressive*, dimension refers to the relationship with oneself, the image that one forms of oneself, and the manner in which one values oneself. This dimension is qualified with the criterion of authenticity. A pedagogic counsellor is authentic when he can take responsibility for his actions, when his actions correspond with the (ideal) image that he has formed of himself. A pedagogic counsellor who can fully identify with the ideas and actions of the team does not experience a discrepancy in his self-image and his actions. His actions are authentic. It is a different case when, for example, the pedagogic counsellor has great doubts about the management of an auto-mutilating person, but continues supporting the approach in his conversations with the parents. He shuts out the parents' criticism, and masks his own doubts. In this case, there is no authenticity in his actions.

With use of the criteria, "skilful", "intimate", and "authentic", one can evaluate the quality of the care of professionals such as pedagogic counsellors. To do this, let us return to the case study.

5. EXPERIENCE OF MEANING AND QUALITY OF CARE

How did the pedagogic counsellor come to a crisis in the experience of meaning? My tentative answer was that his care was not tuned into Frank's changing needs. On the basis of the three criteria for quality (skilful, mutual, and authentic), I will now fine-tune my answer.

5.1. The Technical Dimension: Skilful

The group leaders considered Steven a skilful pedagogic counsellor. They valued his practical advice. He understood the needs of a child whose visual and motor abilities are declining. He made an educated decision about adjusting Frank's communication notebook, and proposed a well thought out plan to keep his mobility at an optimal level. He stayed on top of carrying out the plan. However, when Frank's condition started deteriorating more rapidly, and he started growing more dependent, the pedagogic counsellor became unsure of himself. Frank could now do so little by himself that he had become dependent on the physical care of others. The pedagogic counsellor believed his physical care to be more the group leaders' specialty. He was not able to contribute to this. His role was changing from being the do-er to leaving the work to others. He became less and less actively involved.

This could be explained in a positive manner: he was wise to pull back at the right time. Yet, there is reason to qualify the pulling-back of the pedagogic counsellor as a lack of skill. In the new situation, it became evident that the pedagogic counsellor only understood one type of care need: the need to help enhance Frank's abilities. When there is nothing left to develop, the pedagogic counsellor was left with empty hands. He was not able to signal Frank's greatest needs in a period of deterioration: help in breaking through the increasing isolation, support in the sadness of being less capable, and support in Frank's fear of his increasing seizure activity.

In conclusion, the pedagogic counsellor was skilful in promoting Frank's independence, but lacked skill in understanding his further care needs.

5.2. The Relational Dimension: Mutuality

Frictions in the technical dimension should not be disassociated from the relational dimension in the work of the pedagogic counsellor. During the first years, the pedagogic counsellor was closely involved with Frank. They had frequent contact, beyond what could be expected from a pedagogic counsellor supporting seven different homes. The pedagogic counsellor acted mutually. He built up a trusting relationship with Frank: they "talked" with each other by means of the communication notebook, they went on walks, and at mealtime they sat face to face. There was a strong bond between them. When Frank was ill, the pedagogic counsellor called to inquire about him. Their mutuality benefited not only Frank, but Steven as well. It was clear that Steven's contact with Frank was emotionally meaningful to him.

This only made it more shocking when the pedagogic counsellor visited Frank less frequently as his condition started deteriorating, and as he became nearly completely dependent on those around him. Steven's argument that he was not needed as much appears to be more a rationalization of his own powerlessness than a justification of his decreasing involvement. It is worth noting that the group leaders did not blame Steven for not contributing to Frank's care plan, but that they did blame him for his absence. They did not criticize his skills. They blamed the pedagogic counsellor for writing Frank off as just another "case". In other words, they criticized his lack of mutuality.

The absence of the pedagogic counsellor was the result of his inability to commit himself to an increasingly ill child. He could not handle the child's suffering. His spontaneous, trusted approach faltered. His disposition had changed. Yet, the child had not left his thoughts. He worried about him while playing with his own children, and compared Frank with his own son who was about the same age. However, he did not know how to give shape to his concerns. The reasons become clear when we look at the expressive dimension of his actions.

5.3. Expressive Dimension: Authenticity

The expressive dimension of the pedagogic counsellor's work concerns his image of himself, and the way in which he values himself. When self-image and actions correspond, the work of the pedagogic counsellor is authentic. For Steven, this was certainly the case in the first year of his contact with Frank. His approach to working with Frank was successful, and he was valued by the group leaders. His work style fit perfectly with his image of the ideal: to be a practical pedagogic counsellor, closely involved with the daily life of people with mental retardation, and to have good team-work with the group leaders.

When Frank's abilities were starting to decline, however, this idealistic image became pressured. The pedagogic counsellor became less successful in acting in accordance with his image of the ideal. He did not know what more he could do for Frank and the group leaders. He found it difficult to be confronted with a seriously ill child. The child could not meet his image of the ideal: "to help people with mental retardation be as independent as possible." His self-image also formed a roadblock to being able to adjust to the changing circumstances: "this is not the work of a pedagogic counsellor, but is better suited for the group leadership." This is how the pedagogic counsellor came to distance himself from Frank as well as from the group leaders. He continued acting in accordance with his idealistic image and his self-image. In that light, he was authentic. What he gained by this choice is that he did not have to face the fact that he, by holding onto his image of the ideal, had failed as a pedagogic counsellor. His bubble was burst by the fiery criticism of the group leaders, who blamed him for failing them. Their reaction was intense because they had known him differently: he had been so involved, and now had become so indifferent. The pedagogic counsellor was confronted with the fact that others did not consider his actions to be authentic. The discrepancy between his self-image and the perception of others was for him the breaking point.

6. CRISIS IN THE EXPERIENCE OF MEANING: AN EVALUATION

The actions of the pedagogic counsellor can by typified as skilful, intimate, and authentic. That is, if one looks at the first year and a half of Frank's stay in Westeinde. However, when Frank deteriorated more rapidly, Steven was no longer able to respond skilfully and mutually to the changing needs. The pedagogic counsellor found himself in an impasse. This was coupled with doubts about the meaning of his work and the meaning of the life of children such as Frank.

The breaking point in the experience of meaning of the pedagogic counsellor seems to be the fact that he clutched on to ideals which no longer corresponded to the new situation. The case does not explicitly inform us of the specific ideals which caused the pedagogic counsellor to stumble. Still, some information can be deduced. In my opinion, two ideals played a role in the thoughts and actions of the pedagogic counsellor. These ideals are narrowly entwined, and perhaps are even each other's mirror image.

I would like to refer to the first ideal as the *autonomy-ideal*. The pedagogic counsellor envisioned maximal independence for people with mental retardation. For him, this went beyond a goal that is adjusted according to the given circumstances and possibilities. It was an ideal which clouded his perception, and which shut his eyes for those aspects of Frank's needs that did not match his image of the ideal. As long as he was able to contribute to promoting Frank's independence, the pedagogic counsellor was active and creative. But when he came to the realization that in Frank's case this was an illusion, he pulled out, not giving up his image of the ideal, nor opening it up to discussion.

The second ideal can be identified as the *production ideal*. In the case study, the pedagogic counsellor aimed for a tangible result. His identity as a professional would stand or fall with the success of the treatment plan. As long as Frank made gains, even with the slightest possibility for improvement, Steven gave it his all.

When the care became more custodial, and when (as a matter of speech) production turned into maintenance, he became unsure of what more he could do. He did not know how to resolve the tension between passivity and activity, between living in the "here and now" and focusing on future goals. Mere physical care did not live up to his "production-ideal".

In order to hold on to these ideals, and to not relinquish his vision of the identity of a pedagogic counsellor, he distanced himself from Frank. He wanted to remain authentic, and to do this, he had to pay a high price. By fixating on his ideals, he was no longer able to work skilfully and mutually. He was incapable of substantiating Frank's current needs in an objective manner, let alone being capable of coming up with an adequate answer to his needs. He was not able to entrust himself to Frank, let alone being able to gain the trust of a child that was becoming more and more isolated.

The stagnation in the expressive dimension of the work of the pedagogic counsellor, and its continuation in the technical and relational dimensions of his work, help us to understand why he got "stuck" when Frank deteriorated, and why he began doubting the meaning of his work and the meaning of Frank's life. His own children played an important role in this doubt. They were the living examples of his ideals. Through them, he was face to face with his ideals on a daily basis. By comparing the lives of his children with that of Frank, his doubts were fed, and the gap between the ideal and reality became increasingly great.

7. SELF-EVALUATION

Now that we have come to a greater understanding of the development of the pedagogic counsellor's crisis in the experience of meaning, I will return to the question of what Steven might have done to get out of this impasse. In any case, there should have been a discussion with the group leaders about their team-work and regarding Frank's care plan. Before the pedagogic counsellor initiates this discussion, it is advisable that he first understands himself better. In doing so, he could also seek the advice of a colleague or supervisor. In general lines, I will indicate which subjects should come up in the discussion he has with himself and with others. I will address these in a question format. Since it concerns a self evaluation, I will formulate the questions in the subjective. The questions are based on the group leaders' criticism of the pedagogic counsellor. I will start with the issues that carried the most weight for the group leaders as well as for the pedagogic counsellor.

7.1. Experience of Meaning — Relational Dimension

The greatest complaint of the group leaders was that the pedagogic counsellor had not come to see Frank in three months. They blamed him for pulling out of the "Frank case". The pedagogic counsellor admitted that he had fallen short. His reaction, "you are right," was not enough, however. He owed the group leaders an explanation. The blame of the group leaders concerned the relational dimension of the pedagogic counsellor's work. With this in view, the following questions are of importance:

- Why did I use to visit Frank so frequently, and do I now avoid contact with him? Is this in Frank's best interest, or in my own?
- Why is it so difficult to entrust myself to Frank, like I used to? Is it because he doesn't need this trust as much?
- Why do I hope Frank won't live much longer? Is this for him, or for me?
- Do I doubt the meaning of Frank's life? If so, why do I doubt this now, and not before? Is it because Frank is so ill, and/or because I find it difficult to entrust myself to him?

By considering these questions, the pedagogic counsellor will gain insight into the relational dimension of his actions, particularly regarding the relationship between his disposition and the way in which he experiences meaning in Frank's life. With this understanding, he can begin the discussion with the group leaders regarding their reproach that he deserted Frank.

7.2. Experience of Meaning — Expressive Dimension

The group leaders blamed the pedagogic counsellor for leaving them out in the cold. This greatly disappointed them. At first, there had been such good team-work, but as soon as Frank's condition deteriorated, he disappeared. This was not how they knew him. They were no longer sure whether they could depend on him, or what he was all about. Their reproach concerned the expressive dimension of the pedagogic counsellor's actions. With this in view, the following questions are of importance:

- What is important to me in my work? What kind of a pedagogic counsellor do I want to be?
- Is my work style in line with my ideals, particularly in regard to my work with Frank? How does the way it is now compare with how it was when he was doing better?
- What sort of impression would I want the group leaders to have of me? Why has their appreciation of me changed? Do I understand why they believe that I have changed?
- I believe that the physical part of Frank's care is not part of my profession. Now that his needs are mostly custodial, I find that I cannot make a meaningful contribution to his care. Why is this my belief? Is it correct?
- As a pedagogic counsellor, is there anything more I can do for Frank? If so, do I want to?
- Am I willing to talk about this in all openness with the group leaders?

By means of these questions, the pedagogic counsellor can gain insight into the expressive dimension of his actions. The main purpose is for him to gain insight into his motives to hold on to his ideals in changed circumstances. The pedagogic counsellor must make clear to the group leaders whether he can or wants to contribute to carrying out the team care plan for Frank.

7.3. Experience of Meaning — Technical Dimension

The group leaders did not criticize the skill of the pedagogic counsellor. At least, they did not bring it up. It actually was not possible to make a judgment of the technical dimension of his work since the pedagogic counsellor had pulled away from the situation, and was no longer contributing to the team care plan. This lack of involvement was closely associated with his crisis in experiencing meaning in his work. With this in view, the following questions are of importance:

- Under the present circumstances, I find it difficult to entrust myself to Frank. How does this influence the technical dimension of my work? Am I able to make a realistic calculation of his needs, now I don't see him anymore?
- My primary goal in working with people with mental retardation is the promotion of their independence. This is no longer a goal for Frank. Does this mean that, according to my interpretation of a pedagogic counsellor's contribution to the care plan, I have no more input to give? Can it be that, due to my perspective, Frank has needs which I am blind to?
- How can I find out what I could still do for Frank?

By answering these questions, the pedagogic counsellor gains insight into the influence of his disposition and his ideals on the quality of the technical dimension of his work. He might find out that he is very selective in his perception of the situation, there being needs he is not aware of. This insight allows for an opening in the discussion with the group leaders regarding a renewed contribution to Frank's care plan. This way, his doubts about the meaning of his work could be resolved.

8. FOUNDATIONS OF EXPERIENCING MEANING

The experience of meaning of the pedagogic counsellor, Steven, is a good example of the experiences of other care-givers. Those who work with people with mental retardation will, just like the parents, sooner or later be confronted with the large and painful discrepancy between the ideal and reality. Some will run aground. Others will go through the tiresome process of adjusting their ideals, and accepting a reality that is far different from what anyone would have expected or dreamed of. The case study illustrates a breaking point in this process: holding on to ideals that are not appropriate for people with serious limitations. The pedagogic counsellor's norm for defining meaning[3] actually helped bring on a crisis.

We will now move away from the specific circumstances of the case study to discuss, in general terms, a more appropriate norm: the general conditions under which one can experience meaning in the life and care of people with mental retardation. I will do this by means of answering the question of how meaningful experiences come about (generally). What causes us to consider something meaningful? Van Woudenberg gives three possible reasons.[4] One finds something meaningful (1) when it meets a certain goal, (2) when it has value in and of itself, or (3) when one experiences something as a calling. These reasons assume varying norms for defining meaning. I will explore these successively, and will assess whether they are appropriate.

8.1. Meeting a Certain Goal

One can experience something as meaningful because it contributes to meeting a certain goal. A student who wants to travel and is in need of money will experience a summer-job as meaningful, even if he finds the work boring. In the same way, an author who is unable to find a publisher for his book will at some point stop writing, since he sees no meaning in writing a book that will stay on his shelf.

Raising children is by definition a purposeful task. The meaning of child-rearing lies in helping, challenging, and stimulating children toward becoming mature and independent. The energy put into this is time well spent. The dominating factor in experiencing meaning in child-rearing is its goal, especially in a culture where rationality, autonomy, and achievement are highly valued. These ideals function as norms for defining meaning in child-rearing.

The problem is, however, that the ideals are often set so high that a child could never reach them. This is particularly true for children with mental retardation. Following the principle of equality, handicapped children are, just like other children, raised with goals such as emancipation, integration, autonomy, and freedom of choice. To a large extent, these goals are irrealistic. If they can realize these goals at all, it would be in a very limited way. As a result, those who work with children with mental retardation are continually forced to adjust, sometimes even to give up, their goals. What meaning is there in raising a child, when it will never learn how to walk, talk, or play; when it will always remain dependent? When a care-giver is confronted with the limitations of a child with mental retardation, and of himself, he will discover how inappropriate goals put a strain on the experience of meaning in raising this child.

In my opinion, these types of goals (such as autonomy), are a shaky basis for one's experience of meaning. The case study clearly demonstrates this. In order to avoid a misunderstanding, I am not saying that setting care goals is taboo. Against a background of years of patronizing people with mental retardation and of "knowing what is best for them", the goal of "promoting the freedom of choice", does contribute to keeping the care on the right track. Neither do I mean to say that working with a child on a communication program could not be a meaningful experience for the child or the care-giver. Anything which contributes to reaching a goal can be experienced as meaningful. Setting goals in one's work with people with mental retardation can definitely be a norm for defining meaning. But it should never be the only, and certainly not the most fundamental, norm for defining meaning.

8.2. Value in and of Itself

As already indicated in the Introduction, this book considers human life to be valuable *a priori*. Each person's life has intrinsic value, regardless of his or her abilities. It is this value that I consider to be the most important norm for defining meaning in the care for people with mental retardation.

Simply finding meaning or value in someone or something does not obligate anyone. One can consider protection of the environment to be meaningful, and yet not be obligated to be actively involved. In my opinion however, if someone acknowledges that something or someone has meaning, he carries a moral obligation to treat it with care. The value of human life has the character of an imperative. Acknowledging this value obligates us to be actively involved, to care for and help where needed. When it comes to people with mental retardation, coupling value and care is not as easy as it seems. Even when one agrees that their life is valuable, it is not always so easy to discover and experience this value. How do I discover this value? How should I picture this abstract concept in my mind? How is meaning lived out through my actions? Since a lengthy discussion goes beyond the scope of this contribution, I will address these questions in brief.

At the first encounter with a child with mental retardation, the instinctive reaction often is to turn away. Even though one believes in the inherent value of this child's life, this value is not automatically experienced. It seems to be hidden behind a facade of outward features that at first tend to scare a person off. He who tries to break through this facade will realize that it is not possible to discover the meaning of a seriously handicapped child by means of reasoning. This meaning is only found when one is actively involved with the child: in cuddling with, touching, dressing, and feeding the child. Such involvement is both active and passive. Experiencing meaning requires a passive susceptibility to, as well as an active search for, the signs pointing to the meaning of the handicapped child's life.[5]

This brings us to the second question: how should we picture the abstract concept of meaning in our minds? Elsewhere, I have connected the value of human life with their personhood.[6] The concept of personhood touches the core of being human. Being a "person" points to the uniqueness of being human, as well to the special value of one's life. For a human to be a person, it is not required of him to meet certain expectations. It is independent of age, sex, looks, (mental) abilities, achievements, or societal usefulness. Each human being is a person simply because he is.[7] Being a person, each human's life has irreplaceable value and each human's life has meaning.

However, "personhood" does not say everything about being a human. The human being is more than just a person. Better said: he can become more. An inherent part of being a person is the longing for one's personality to grow with its own identity, to share one's life with others, and to experience life to be good and meaningful. I am assuming that all humans have this longing. People, even people with serious multiple handicaps, long for an *identity-in-connectedness* (passively or actively, consciously or unconsciously). This is the longing to be accepted, in relation to others, as well as (in a religious sense) in relation to God. This longing has the character of a postulate: a necessary principle which is not only required, but also wants to be realized. In other words, the longing for identity-in-connectedness is a principle which motivates human interaction, and which must be realized in human relations. All that contributes to this realization is meaningful.

Experience teaches us that not everyone will be able to realize their longing for identity-in-connectedness in the same fashion, nor to the same extent. Herein lies a large gap between people with or without mental retardation. Even so, no human being will be able to realize this longing alone. People cannot go without the attention, the love, and the help of others. This fact carries a clear moral implication. Human personhood makes an appeal to others to help realize the longing for identity-in-connectedness. This appeal is obligating. Being a person implies that the human (with mental retardation) needs to be confirmed in the meaning and value of their life by means of the active involvement of others. Confirming the meaning of another's life is a meaningful action. He who cares for people with mental retardation does meaningful work.

Having said this, I won't need to be lengthy in answering the third question: how is meaning lived out through my actions? To find the meaning, or value, of the life of children (with mental retardation), one should look at their longing for identity-in-connectedness. It is the responsibility of the care-givers to respond to their longing in a meaningful (a skilful, intimate, and authentic) way.

The case study demonstrates how one should not have too romantic a picture of the form this takes in the actual care of people with mental retardation. Finding meaning in the life of a child with severe mental retardation does not happen by itself, but requires an intensive search for the identity, and the uniqueness of the child, and for the possibilities of having contact with the child. But even a lengthy and intensive involvement is not a guarantee for understanding the child's needs. It is possible that one's involvement leads to nowhere, and that not the least bit of meaning is experienced. There are, as we saw, situations in which meaning is initially experienced, but later dissipates. Even so, the intrinsic value of the child's life (as a norm for defining meaning) will always remain.

8.3. Calling

Van Woudenberg points out yet a third reason for finding something meaningful, namely the sense of being called to something. The concept of "calling" can be understood in a religious, as well as a secular way.

In the *religious* sense, we talk about a Divine calling, by which a person finds his purpose. This can be thought of as one's eternal destiny, but also as a fulfillment of a certain life task or a special mission. Heeding this calling, and doing what God asks, is a source of experiencing meaning. In his historical account of the genesis of the care of people with mental retardation in the Netherlands, Jak gives some poignant examples.[8] In the nineteenth century, several teachers, pastors, and priests felt called to start "Homes of Mercy", by which the foundation was laid for the present-day health care programs for people with mental retardation. In many countries, the care for the "least" in society got started by those who sensed a calling.

Being called, as a norm for defining meaning, plays an important role in the christian living communities of l'Arche, which were founded during the past thirty years. Considering the theme of this contribution, it is interesting to note that Nouwen, one of the most well known representatives of l'Arche, understood his calling as a commission to not only care for and give to people with handicaps, but above all to receive from them, by simply being open to the "enormous riches of their presence in society".[9] It is this calling that Nouwen considers the most important source of experiencing meaning in the care for people with mental retardation.

A calling may also have a *secular* character. In this case, one does not experience a Divine calling which comes from without, but rather feels an inner calling. Through a strong inner urging, one decides to take on a certain task, such as caring for people with mental retardation. Once on the job, this calling can function as a norm for defining meaning. This can help a pedagogic counsellor when he feels stuck in the care of a man or woman with mental retardation. When he feels discouraged, he can draw new inspiration from the thought of why he once felt dedicated to this work. Remembering his sense of calling will give him a renewed perspective in the meaning of his work.

9. SUMMARY

Under which conditions can the life of people with mental retardation and their care be experienced as meaningful? This was the central theme of this contribution. To summarize the answer, in a care-giver's work, meaning can be defined by three norms: the realization of goals in one's work with people with mental retardation; the acknowledgement of the intrinsic value of their lives; and the calling to work in their care. The second norm is fundamental for experiencing meaning. The first is important, but not decisive. The third norm is, especially under difficult circumstances, a source of inspiration.

NOTES

1 In the Netherlands, pedagogic counsellors play a central role in the care for people with mental retardation. Their most important task is developing, carrying out, and evaluating the individual care plans of their clients. In doing this, they work hand in hand with a.o. group leaders, who provide the daily care in group homes or day-care centers. It is the pedagogic counsellor's job to provide guidance to the group leaders in their tasks. In the Netherlands, pedagogic counsellors receive a university education, and usually receive additional schooling beyond their degree.

2 See a.o. P.A. de Ruyter, "Pedagogische hulpverleningsvisies" (Concepts of Pedagogic Care), in R. de Groot, K. Doornbos, J.D. van der Ploeg, and P.A. De Ruyter (eds.), *Handboek Orthopedagogiek* (The Pedagogic Counsellor's Manual). Groningen: Wolters-Noordhoff, rubriek 3104, (1993), pp. 1-31; P.A. de Ruyter and J. Stolk, "Wanneer is het hulpverlenend handelen goed genoeg?" (When Is Assistance Good Enough?), in H. Kars (ed.), *Ernstig probleemgedrag bij zwakzinnige mensen* (Severely Problematic Behavior of People with Mental Retardation). Houten: Bohn Stafleu Van Loghum, 1995, pp. 35-54.

3 The concept of a norm for defining meaning is developed in the Introduction.

4 R. van Woudenberg, *Gelovend denken. Inleiding tot een christelijke filosofie* (Faith and Reason: An Introduction to a Christian Philosophy). Amsterdam: Buijten en Schipperheijn, 1992, pp. 193ff.

5 The contributions of Young and De Ruyter (chapters 1 and 11) illustrate this in more detail.

6 See J. Stolk, "Die Frage nach dem Wert des Lebens geistig behinderter Kinder" (On the Value of Life of Children with Mental Retardation), in W. Thimm *et al.* (eds.), *Ethische Aspekte der Hilfen für Behinderte* (Ethical Aspects of Caring for People with a Handicap). Marburg, Germany: Lebenshilfe Deutschland, 1989, pp. 184-213; J. Stolk, "Geistig behindert mit dem Verlangen auch jemand zu sein" (People with Mental Retardation Longing for Identity), in J. Stolk and M.J.A. Egberts (eds.), *Über die Würde geistig behinderter Menschen, Zwischen Verlangen und Wirklichkeit* (The Dignity of People with Mental Retardation: Between Dream and Reality). Marburg, Germany: Lebenshilfe Deutschland, 1990, pp. 5-34.

7 The concept of personhood as described here, can be typified as 'static.' Personhood is considered an ontological quality. One can also view the personhood of humans in a dynamic way: personhood is the product of human development. This conception is bound to certain conditions. A child becomes a person only once it has met a certain developmental level. The choice for using a static or dynamic concept for personhood has important moral implications for the care of people with mental retardation. This comes to light in the discussion regarding the right to protection of the life of seriously handicapped newborns, in which the concept of personhood plays a crucial role. See G. Antor and U. Bleidick, *Recht auf Leben, Recht auf Bildung. Aktuelle Fragen der Behindertenpädagogik* (Right to Life, Right to Education: On Educating People with Handicaps). Heidelberg, Germany: Schindele Publishers, 1995. My choice to use the static concept of personhood must be seen in light of this discussion. *Cf.* J. Stolk, "The concept of the person: valuing the life of severely handicapped babies," in J.M. Berg *et al.*, *Report on the European workshop "Bio-ethics and Mental Handicap".* Utrecht: Bishop Bekkers Foundation, 1992, pp. 117-28.

8 See Th. Jak, *Huizen van Barmhartigheid. Zorg voor zwakzinnigen in Nederland in de tweede helft van de negentiende eeuw, met bijzondere aandacht voor 's Heeren Loo* (Homes of Mercy: Care of People with Mental Retardation in the Second Half of the 19th Century). Amersfoort: Vereniging 's Heeren Loo, 1993.

9 Henri Nouwen interviewed by Wolterink in *Contactblad Philadelphia*, Vol. 177, (1994), pp. 6-8.

INDEX

NAMES

SUBJECTS

CONTRIBUTORS

Theo A. Boer, Ph.D., is a researcher at the Center for Bio-ethics and Health Law, Utrecht University, Secretary of Studies of the Christian Association of Health Care Facilities. He also teaches Christian ethics at the faculty of Divinity of Utrecht University, the Netherlands.

Gerendina (Diny) van Bruggen, M.D., is a paediatrician, with 15 years of practice in Dutch hospitals and 10 years of working in developing countries and refugee camps.

Ulrich Eibach, Ph.D., is a professor of Medical Ethics, University of Bonn, Germany, and hospital chaplain at the Academic Hospital in Bonn.

Ralph Evers, M.L., M.D., is Rabbi of the Dutch Israelite Denomination and Dean of the Dutch Israelite Seminary

Stanley M. Hauerwas, Ph.D., is a professor of Theological Ethics, Duke University, North Carolina, USA.

Henk Kars, Ph.D., is a psychologist and former senior staff worker at "Eemeroord" a center for people with mental retardation, Baarn, the Netherlands.

Johannes (Hans) S. Reinders, Ph.D., is a professor of Theological Ethics, and a professor of Ethics concerning the care for people with mental retardation, Free University, Amsterdam, the Netherlands.

Pieter A. de Ruyter, Ph.D., is a professor of Special Pedagogics, Free University Amsterdam, the Netherlands.

Ruth Seldenrijk, M.D., is a biophysicist and senior staff worker at the Department of Research and Development of the Dutch association of care facilities, 's Heeren Loo, Amersfoort, the Netherlands.

Joop Stolk, Ph.D., is an associate professor of Special Pedagogics, Free University, Amsterdam, the Netherlands.

Frances Young, Ph.D., is a professor of Theology, University of Birmingham, England.